Springer Series on the Teaching of Nursing

Diane O. McGivern, RN, PhD, FAAN, Series Editor
New York University

Advisory Board: *Ellen Baer, PhD, RN, FAAN; Carla Mariano, EdD, RN, AHN-C, FAAIM; Janet A. Rodgers, PhD, RN, FAAN; Alice Adam Young, PhD, RN*

About the Authors

Jeanne M. Novotny, **PhD**, **RN**, **FAAN**, is currently dean and professor at the Fairfield University School of Nursing. She received her bachelor's and master of science degrees in nursing from Ohio State University and her PhD from Kent State University. Her career encompasses more than three decades of leadership in nursing education and administration. Dr. Novotny came to Fairfield University from the University of Virginia in 2001. She has done international work in Mexico, Chile, and Zimbabwe. Dr. Novotny holds a certificate from the Institute for Management and Leadership in Education at Harvard University and is an evaluator for the Commission on Collegiate Nursing Education. Dr. Novotny has clinical expertise in pediatric nursing and nursing leadership and has numerous scholarly publications, presentations, and consultations to her credit.

Mary T. Quinn Griffin, **PhD**, **RN**, is an assistant professor of nursing at the Frances Payne Bolton School of Nursing at Case Western Reserve University. She received her M.Ed. degree from Dublin University's Trinity College and both her MSN and her PhD in nursing from Case Western Reserve University. Dr. Quinn Griffin has over 20 years' experience in nursing education in Ireland and the United States, having taught across a variety of nursing programs, as well as experience in educational administration. She has completed studies in the Web-Based Genetics Institute of the Genetics Program for Nursing at Cincinnati Children's Hospital and developed strategies for integrating genetics into the curriculum. Currently, her research focus is in genetics and ethics related to genetic research. She is a faculty associate of the Center for Genetic Research Ethics and Law (CGREAL) at Case Western Reserve University, an interdisciplinary Center for Excellence in Ethical, Legal and Social Implications Research funded by the National Institutes of Health. Dr. Quinn Griffin has a degree in molecular genetics from Georgetown University. Dr. Quinn Griffin is an active member of Sigma Theta Tau International.

A Nuts-and-Bolts Approach to Teaching Nursing

Third Edition

Jeanne M. Novotny, PhD, RN, FAAN

Mary T. Quinn Griffin, PhD, RN

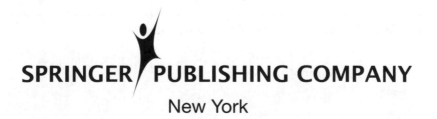

SPRINGER PUBLISHING COMPANY

New York

Springer Publishing Company, Inc.
11 West 42nd Street
New York, NY 10036

Acquisitions Editor: Sally J. Barhydt
Managing Editor: Mary Ann McLaughlin
Production Editor: Emily Johnston
Cover design by Joanne E. Honigman
Typeset by Apex Publishing

07   08   09   10/   5   4   3   2

Library of Congress Cataloging-in-Publication Data

Novotny, Jeanne.
    Nuts-and-bolts approach to teaching nursing.— 3rd ed. / Jeanne M. Novotny, Mary T. Quinn Griffin.
        p. ; cm. — (Springer series on the teaching of nursing)
    Rev. ed. of: A nuts-and-bolts approach to teaching nursing / Victoria Schoolcraft. 2nd ed. c2000.
    Includes bibliographical references and index.
    ISBN 0-8261-6602-4
    ISBN 978-0-8261-6602-9
    1. Nursing—Study and teaching. I. Griffin, Mary T. Quinn. II. Schoolcraft, Victoria. Nuts-and-bolts approach to teaching nursing. III. Title. IV. Series: Springer series on the teaching of nursing (Unnumbered)
    [DNLM: 1. Education, Nursing. 2. Teaching—methods. WY 18 N945n 2006]
RT90.N68 2006   2006013397
610.73071'1-—dc22   CIP

Printed in the United States of America by Bang Printing

Contents

List of Tables

Preface

To start with, make sure you have noticed that this book is *not* subtitled "Everything You Need to Know to Teach Nursing." It is meant to be, as it is called, the "nuts and bolts" of how to teach, a survival manual for those who are teaching for the first time and need a reference book, or for those who will eventually work on expanding their knowledge through formal course work. It is also an excellent refresher for faculty members reentering full- and part-time positions. This book is not meant to replace a sound graduate educational program, and so if you are searching for something scholarly and theoretical, stop here!

This book will be valuable to faculty teaching nursing students in any type of program, from practical nursing through a master's course. Faculty members will find some chapters to be more helpful than others in particular teaching situations. For example, if you work with practical nursing students, you do need to consider the variables in assigning patients and supervising students' clinical practice. However, it is unlikely that you would need to plan a seminar course or require complex written assignments.

The information in this book will be of greatest use to faculty members teaching undergraduate students in associate-degree and baccalaureate programs. Your expectations of students will vary with the educational level. For example, you would not expect a second-year associate degree student to complete the complex assignments that you might expect from a fourth-year baccalaureate student. We have tried to indicate factors to help you discriminate which assignments would be appropriate for which students.

Because of the practical, hands-on nature of this book, we have avoided the theoretical. Lists of resources for further reading have been provided for those interested in pursuing specific topics in more depth, but our intention has been to follow Victoria Schoolcraft's practical aspects of teaching and to draw on our own experiences and our colleagues' experiences. Although the chapter titles reflect the previous editions of this book, the contents and suggested readings have been thoroughly revised and updated.

In publishing this third edition of *A Nuts-and-Bolts Approach to Teaching Nursing,* we wish to say thank you to Victoria Schoolcraft, the original author of this book and this teaching concept, for the way that she taught faculty to work with students. Although she died before the second edition was published, her voice has been preserved in these pages. Her legacy will thrive and continue because faculty responsibilities in the transmission of knowledge intertwined with the roles of practice and research will only become more important in the future.

We would like to acknowledge the contributions of the following students in the Doctor of Nursing Practice program at Frances Payne Bolton School of Nursing at Case Western Reserve University, specifically in the teaching practicum course:

Jeanette Cheshire
Moreen Donahue
Kathleen A. Ennis
Kelly Jones
Darlene Mathis
Kathleen Meyers
Virginia Peterson
Irene Piazza
Deborah Rodell
Eva W. Stephens
Anne Swallow

It is our hope that you will find the book helpful and encouraging. We also hope that you will love teaching nursing students as much as we do!

Jeanne M. Novotny
Mary T. Quinn Griffin

1

Making Clinical Assignments

If history has any message for nursing, it is that students need the clinical setting to apply the knowledge that is gained from classes, readings, group discussions, skills labs, and other learning experiences. If you ask students or graduates what they would change about the nursing curriculum, the majority would proclaim, "More clinical!" This element of the curriculum is essential to students' increase in self-confidence, development of critical thinking skills, and transformation into professional nurses.

Self-confidence as a nurse cannot be learned in the classroom. Therefore, gaining self-confidence is one of the most important aspects of the clinical experience. Only by trying and mastering new skills can students overcome feelings of incompetence and gain the self-assurance necessary to develop the inner security needed to make sound clinical judgments in the real world.

Once faculty members determine how much time will be spent in the clinical setting, the next step is to determine how to make the most of this time. The key to this process is selecting increasingly challenging patients for students, so that over time, each student gets as much clinical experience and as broad a learning opportunity as possible. To maximize the likelihood of this outcome, each selection of a patient must provide the students with the opportunity to apply the theoretical information gained from the classroom and other assignments. Every hour in the clinical setting must contribute to the students' ability to learn and master the expected content. This is made possible by the careful selection of patients whose care delivery reinforces weekly learning objectives.

GOALS

The principal goal for the clinical experience is to provide the opportunity for the application of theory and the validation of skills. The most effective clinical settings provide students with an opportunity to practice their psychomotor skills, refine their critical thinking abilities, and develop their psychosocial skills with actual patients and their families. This process increases students' feelings of confidence and self-esteem and promotes achievement of expected competencies.

TOOLS

Course Objectives

The main factor to consider when determining which patients to assign to students is the course objectives. If the course objectives relate to caring for patients with "simple disruptions in their physical health status," assign patients who match that description as closely as possible. Because it is difficult in this era to find patients who have simple disruptions in health status, close supervision and support may be required until the students' level of comfort reaches an acceptable level. Efforts should be made to assign beginning students in a manner that does not overwhelm them. In an early clinical course, the faculty member may have no choice but to assign patients with complex problems. The focus of the student actions, however, will be directed toward management of basic needs.

Clinical Objectives

In addition to course objectives, faculty should develop detailed clinical objectives that specify the expectations for performance and that identify the process of evaluation. These objectives flow from the overall course objectives and link application expectations to knowledge-development components. For example, identify at least three nursing interventions for a patient at risk for skin breakdown related to immobility; the clinical objectives should state exactly how students would be evaluated when performing psychosocial and psychomotor skills. An acceptable level of competence or skill performance also should be identified.

Student Learning Needs

Course and clinical objectives relate to the learning planned for all the students. In order for each student's needs to be met, however, some modification of additional learning experiences may be required. Differences may exist in the speed at which students learn and in the learning techniques they find most useful. The ability to perform at a certain level may be attained much more quickly by some students. Rather than holding these students back, assign patients whose care permits the students to accomplish new or expanded objectives.

Give each student as much variety as possible in the types of patients assigned. This includes providing for different medical and nursing diagnoses as well as a variety of demographic parameters. Keep track of this information on a card or notebook with anecdotal notes.

For example, this record may reflect the efforts made to assign patients with a focus on mobility in the first week. In the second week, a notation could be made about the shift of the focus to problems with gastrointestinal disturbances. The third week might focus on surgical patients, and the fourth would perhaps reflect an assignment related to elderly patients. Such a record helps make certain that a student is not repeatedly assigned the same kind of patient. It also helps faculty keep track of the opportunities that students have to give medications, to perform discharge planning, and to do anything else that meets the students' learning needs for achieving clinical objectives.

NUTS AND BOLTS

Choosing Patients

Availability

Regardless of what kinds of patients are desired for students' assignments, faculty can only work with the patients who are actually present. Some patients in the census will not be suitable for a variety of reasons. Also, faculty from other nursing programs or other levels within the same school may be competing for the same patients to assign. While considering what patents are available, the faculty member has to decide the most important things for the student to accomplish and must determine which patient's care can provide the best experience to achieve that. Faculty may have to give students a patient much like one assigned in the past, but with direction to focus on something new or more involved than before.

Staff Consultation

The nurse manager is indispensable in determining which patients to assign to students. Nurse managers often have information that may encourage or discourage faculty decision-making about assignments. Faculty also will have to determine how best to work with the unit manager, while focusing on meeting the individual students' learning needs. To do this, faculty should meet with staff prior to the beginning of the rotation to get to know them personally and to hear their expectations for interacting with students and faculty. Negotiate with the manager how patient selection will be made. Everything possible should be done to foster collegial relationships with nursing staff and other health care professionals in the setting. Some nurses on the units will love working with students and will bend over backward to ensure that the learning experience is an excellent one. On the other hand, some nurses do not enjoy working with students, and they may convey this perspective to you directly or indirectly. If you are a newcomer, try to rely more on those who like working with students. As you become more comfortable, work on building better relationships with the others and on helping them to understand the short- and long-term benefits of interacting regularly with students.

Provide the nurse manager with copies of the objectives that pertain to the clinical experience. Post a list of things the students are prepared to do, and identify those tasks they can complete either independently or with assistance. This will remind staff about the types of experiences students are seeking and about what aspects of care the students will be expected to perform during the clinical rotation.

Negotiate with the nurses concerning when to ask for staff input. Some nurses prefer to provide a list that has narrowed down the patient-assignment options. Others will prefer that faculty make some selections and will then provide feedback as needed. Plenty of time should be allowed for consulting with staff when making assignments. In addition, faculty members must be flexible and must accommodate unpredictable or uncontrollable demands on staff time. After faculty and the staff have worked together for a while, adjustments may be made to the original arrangements. Over time, a more give-and-take approach may be possible.

Avoiding Overloading

In a setting that has many student groups, patients may become overwhelmed by the number of students assigned to take care of them. Even good students may be taxing to patients. Because students are slower and less certain, they often inadvertently delay or prolong the tasks they do in providing care. This should be considered when making assignments, and periods of nonstudent assignment may be necessary to allow patients a short-term break.

Multiple Assignments

Although it is appropriate and often a useful experience for more than one student to care for a patient, this may be stressful for the patient. One way to deal with this is to assign one student to do the physical care, another to prepare and pass medications and complete procedures such as dressing changes, and a third to develop a plan of care. This process helps students learn collaborative behaviors, and they often find the experience supportive and rewarding. It also facilitates the sharing of students' learning experiences in the postclinical conference.

Assignments

It is not appropriate to post patient assignments, which would violate the patients' right to privacy. The student needs only to know what unit the patient is assigned to and to then make a visit to meet the patient and review the chart.

In some instances, students are unable to or are not expected to complete extensive patient-care planning prior to the clinical day or days. This is particularly true if the student must travel a considerable distance to reach the clinical area. Nonetheless, the faculty member may still want the student to be familiar with the patient. In that case, these expectations should be made clear at the beginning of the course, and all students should be held to the same standards regarding preparation for a patient assignment.

Student Involvement

As students progress in a course or through the curriculum, they may want to become more involved in selecting patients. One way to accomplish this is to ask students if there are particular types of patients with whom they want to work and to then make your assignments accordingly. In doing so, faculty should be certain that the students select patients who meet the course and clinical objectives and individual learning needs. The faculty member could make a list of patients greater in number than the number of students and allow students to select from that list. Before trying this option, be sure the nurse manager on the unit understands and agrees with this approach.

Patient Involvement

To paraphrase Shakespeare, "To ask or not to ask the patient, that is the question." The primary reason to ask a patient about assigning a student is the existence of some reason to think the patient might be reluctant to accept a student. For example, consider that a patient asked that a certain student no longer be assigned to take care of her. When asked about the reason for the request, the patient responded that this had more to do with that particular student than with something generally pertaining to nursing students. In this case, the patient was willing to try a different student.

Some faculty members who seem to have no reservations about assigning female students to male patients have qualms about assigning male students to female patients. Although some assumptions in this area may be based on bias, it is true that some female patients have concerns about male students being involved with their nursing care.

One way to deal with the assignment of male students is to discuss with the student the possibility of being rejected because of gender. Help the student see the importance of being direct and conveying confidence when making the initial introduction to the assigned patient. A female student or nurse may sometimes find it appropriate to request assistance from a male colleague in giving care to a male patient. In any case, discuss this with the patient. All male and female nurses need to understand and be able to provide complete care for both male and female patients.

Other Settings

Psychiatric Units

A typical approach in most programs is to assign one psychiatric patient to each student for the development of an ongoing relationship. Make sure that staff members are clear about what students need to accomplish, and clarify those expectations and any restrictions that may affect the goals of the experience.

Community Health

The pattern for assignments in community health is determined by the appropriate focus for a beginning practitioner in this area. One belief is that the focus should be on traditional public health, which concentrates on the promotion of wellness for populations. Another view of nursing in the community looks at care for individuals and families who require care on different levels of prevention and who are outside acute care institutions. This would include the care of people who have primary prevention needs, such as pregnant women and their families and children, for whom care involves promoting normal growth and development. Nursing in the community also includes caring for people in their homes who were cared for in acute care settings in the recent past. In the latter example, the care is comparable to medical-surgical nursing in the home rather than in the hospital.

Nonpatient Assignments

In some situations, it is warranted to assign students to do something other than total patient care for one or two patients. In making this decision, faculty should consider whether such an option meets objectives for clinical experience. No matter how much a student would like to tag along with the phlebotomist all day, this may not be a good use of clinical time. On the other hand, such an activity may give the student a perspective on a different pattern for delivering care. Whether the activity meets the course objectives should be a determining factor.

When deciding, faculty should look at the quality of the experience in light of the amount of time spent. In order to maximize the use of such an experience, consider giving the student a particular focus for observation. After completing the experience, the student should share with other students what was learned from the focused experience. The student could also be asked to discuss the interpersonal components of the interactions as well as the motor skills involved.

If there are specific deficits in a student's patient-care experiences, rectify the problem by assigning the student to complete certain tasks for a patient rather than provide total care. For example, if students need opportunities to give injections, this could be the focus for the day.

Assignments for short or observational experiences can help to maximize the student's use of clinical time when patients are discharged early or other unforeseen interruptions interfere with the regular pattern of assignments. When this occurs, faculty should expect the student to think through how these experiences relate to the overall clinical component. This may include sharing the experience during a clinical conference or at least discussing it with faculty.

Evaluating the Process

Midway through and at the end of the course, faculty should evaluate the processes used to assign patients to students, the usefulness of the assignments for meeting course objectives, and the students' assessment of the assignment process and its learning effectiveness. Discussions with students and the unit staff and leadership will help clarify where improvements can be made for the future and which experiences were the most beneficial for the student.

Encouraging students to keep a reflections log that summarizes each day's learning experience and the way in which the patient assignments facilitated the learning may be useful for an ongoing review of assignment adequacy. A review of each day's assignment sheet and faculty's anecdotal notes also will provide useful information about how well or poorly the assignment process worked. Using these combined data can be helpful when negotiating possible changes in the assignment process with unit staff and leadership. In all cases, feedback should be provided about the ways in which the students learn best and about how the learning environment might be enhanced for the future.

FINAL WORDS

Clinical assignments are one of the unique features of nursing education. The clinical setting allows students to practice skills and to gain the confidence they need for practicing as professional nurses. When patient assignment is done well, students, patients, and staff benefit through the students' increased awareness of the diversity of patients seen and the similarities inherent in a wide range of patient situations.

FURTHER READING

Jackson, D. & Mannix, J. (2001). Clinical nurses as teachers: Insights from students of nursing in their first semester of study. *Journal of Clinical Nursing, 10,* 270–277.

Scanlan, J. M. (2001). Learning clinical teaching: Is it magic? *Nursing and Health Care Perspectives, 22,* 240–246.

2

Supervising a Clinical Group

When thinking about supervising students in the clinical area, start by reflecting about personal experiences and feelings. Most people teach as they were taught. If you had a stern clinical instructor who made you feel uncomfortable and on the spot, you may believe that was the right way to approach teaching. After all, you turned out pretty well, did you not?

Although a little anxiety may enhance a student's perceptions and ability to learn, too much is immobilizing and counterproductive. One of the most difficult tasks is achieving the right balance between the roles of the caring faculty member and the concerned nurse. The caring faculty member tries to help students learn in a protected situation. The concerned nurse tries to monitor the impact of student care on patients and makes certain the patients are not inconvenienced or hurt by novices. Keep in mind that even the clumsiest, least dedicated students do not intend to hurt anyone, and of course, sometimes even the most enthusiastic and dedicated students make mistakes.

The clinical area is the crucible where the students combine knowledge with application. It is the sine qua non of nursing education. As a nursing educator, it is your responsibility to help students get all they can out of what is a relatively limited experience.

GOALS

Effective supervision of students in the clinical area should foster meaningful learning experiences and ensure safe care for patients or clients.

TOOLS

Course Objectives

The course objectives provide the groundwork for what the students will get out of the clinical experience. If the course is a beginning course in the curriculum, do not expect students to be responsible for complex aspects of patient care. However, even if the course objectives are the most basic, patients may still have complex problems. When supervising students, the clinical instructor is responsible for determining what the students can and cannot do safely. If there are aspects of patient care the students cannot perform, negotiate with the nurse manager who will be responsible for this.

Course objectives pertaining to clinical are often very general, but they should give some indication about the type of patient and the complexity of care with which the student will be concerned. For example, in a basic nursing course, an objective might be: "Identify and implement comfort measures for patients with the following conditions." In a more advanced course, the following objective might be included: "Plan and implement care for patients with multiple system failures."

Clinical Objectives

General course objectives may be detailed into clinical objectives for students to accomplish by the end of the semester. Some faculty members even specify objectives for each week. Most faculty report that it is easier to deal with general clinical objectives rather than to try to set objectives for each week, given that general objectives can be more easily adapted to the patient population. However, when working with beginning students, focus on the steps in the nursing process. When students are learning to use the process, weekly objectives can be written to specify when the students are supposed to focus on each step.

Following are some examples of specific conditions that could be considered regarding a variation on the potential course objective discussed earlier. Identify and implement comfort measures for patients with the following simple medical or surgical problems:

- Limited mobility
- Dermatological disorder
- Outpatient surgical procedure

Following are examples of clinical objectives related to the more advanced course objective "Plan and implement care for patients with multiple system failures":

- Give comprehensive care for a patient with failures of at least two systems.
- Care for a patient who is being monitored by at least one type of device.
- Identify the principal effects of the major drugs used with patients in cardiovascular distress.

Guidelines for Clinical Activities

Rather than objectives, give students guidelines for what they are to accomplish, such as when they must turn in nursing-care plans, when drug cards are to be used, and when they are scheduled to observe a surgical procedure. Written assignments in conjunction with clinical should be handled in the same way as other assignments in terms of their description, submission requirements, and criteria for evaluation.

Nursing-Care Plans

Nursing-care plans are a standard feature of the clinical experience. However, there is much diversity in care-plan formats. It is beyond the scope of this book to deal with the nuances of the nursing process and care plans, but here is a list of some factors to consider in your approach to using care plans:

- Be consistent with the format used by other faculty in your program.
- Be consistent with the theoretical and conceptual values of your curriculum.
- Be consistent with the texts and other readings the students have, or make it clear where and when care plans should vary from those resources.
- Be explicit about what is expected within each step of the plan.
- Match your expectations with the level of the student.
- Be realistic about the amount of information students can read, comprehend, and reorganize into a care-plan format in the amount of time

allowed. Give minimum and maximum limits on length, depth, and breadth.

- Give clear criteria for the evaluation of care plans and how they contribute to the clinical grade.
- Give ample feedback to help students learn from working out the plans.

Some faculty members expect students to start formulating their care plans before starting the clinical day. These care plans would include the initial parts of the nursing process and provide students with a foundation for the day's activities. Whenever possible, give the student sufficient information prior to the beginning of the clinical day. However, because the patient population changes rapidly, often this is not possible.

In some situations, students are not able to go to the clinical area for a planning period prior to the start of clinical. In this case, give them some information about the assigned patients so that they have a general idea of what they will need to do for their patients. They may not start their care plans until after they begin to work with the patients.

Be clear with students about the purpose of the nursing-care plan. If the care plan is a plan for care as well as a report of care given, that should be clear. It is important for students to have the former understanding of the plan as a plan for care in order to make it clear that the care plan is a valid facet of nursing care. If the plan is used only as a report of care given, students see it as merely an assignment that is divorced from the real practice of nursing.

NUTS AND BOLTS

Orienting Students

Orienting Yourself

The school of nursing may assist faculty in getting oriented to the assigned clinical area. If not, arrange this orientation as soon as possible. Find a colleague who has had students in the same agency, especially on the same units where you are assigned. Colleagues can let you in on the way things really work.

Arrange to meet with the staff manager. It is appropriate to start with the nurse manager, but be sure to talk with the other nurses as well. Find out what they expect and want from faculty and students. Are there some things they have been particularly concerned about in the past, when they have had students previously? Share the course objectives with them, and make sure they know how much the students do and do not know. If the nurses will have to provide some aspect of patient care, even if a student is assigned, make sure the nurses understand and agree with what is needed.

Preclinical Meeting

Meet with the students prior to going to the clinical area. During this meeting, cover the general things students can expect from the upcoming clinical rotation. For example, inform them about the kind of unit on which they will be working, the kinds of patients, the staff complement, and what their responsibilities will be. Make sure all the students know how to get where they are going, where to park if they are driving, and where to meet when they get there. Tell them what the expectations are for their attire. Encourage them not to bring personal belongings.

Although your school must provide written policies in a student handbook, it is a good idea to reiterate the pertinent ones every time you start a new clinical rotation. If there is a difference between agency policies and school policies, clarify what the expectations will be for the students. For example, your school may make it optional for students to wear scrubs, but a particular agency may require students to wear uniforms. Make sure the students know whether uniforms are required.

Clinical Orientation

Once at the agency, emphasize the information that students most need to know. More complex tours may come later, but to start with, be sure they can get from the front door to their unit. Show them around the unit, emphasizing the places with which they need to be most familiar. For example, show them the linen room, the utility rooms, the rest rooms, the places where they can leave their personal belongings, and where they may have access to patient charts. Younger, less experienced students are sometimes so anxious about just being in the hospital for the first time that they have trouble remembering much of what happens. Make sure they know how they can find you during clinical time. Introduce them to the staff with whom they will work. If possible, arrange for some time for them to meet with the nurse manager or assistant so that they can learn about general aspects of the unit.

If the clinical rotation is in a clinic or a community setting, some of the same concerns apply. However, if the student is going to be making home visits, that requires a more extensive orientation. Students are usually nervous about visiting clients in their homes. Give them oral and written information to help them feel more secure. Some of the issues to address are listed below.

- Wearing proper attire and identification
- Arranging for a time to visit
- Locating addresses
- Determining what to do if no one is at home
- Not entering a situation that appears unsafe
- Taking a companion along when necessary
- Not transporting clients anywhere in their own car
- Telling clients how they may contact the student

Also prepare a second list that is more detailed and specific to the agency and the location. The issues in the previous list relate to the students' comfort and safety.

Sometimes it is possible for faculty to accompany each student on the first home visit. If there are other activities in which students can participate prior to their first visits, while other students are conducting their first visits, that is probably the optimal way to start. However, in some situations, faculty may not have the luxury of staggering the students' starting visits. Another good way to start is for the students to accompany one of the staff nurses on a visit to the assigned client or family. Because home visits are frequently unsupervised by a faculty member, give the students definite parameters for the content and process of the visits. A typical list of guidelines might include the following principles:

- Limit the times of each visit to no more than one hour.
- Set at least one goal for each visit, but avoid trying to accomplish too much on a visit.
- Let the clients know what the goals are for the visit.
- Encourage the client to ask questions and to help set goals for future visits.
- Clarify for the client when and how goals have been met.

- Include other family members in the interaction when possible and appropriate.
- Use written and pictorial material as well as three-dimensional models to help explain information to clients.
- When collecting data, tell the client what will be done with the information and who will have access to it.
- At the end of the visit, sum up what has been discussed and what the goal of the next visit will be.

Making Assignments

This aspect is covered in detail in chapter 1. Make certain that students know when and where to find information on their assignments. Some faculty expect the students to go to the clinical setting the day before they will give care in order to gather detailed information about the client.

Validating Students' Preparation

It is sometimes difficult to check on each student's preparation before you let him or her get started for the day. Students should share the high points of their patients' care in a preclinical conference before they start. As the day goes by, look for opportunities to talk with each student in more depth. Some faculty members expect the students to hand over the beginning of their care plans before they get started.

Occasionally a student is unprepared. If it is the first time this has happened, send the student to the library to get prepared and give responsibility for the patient's care back to the staff until the student is ready. Students who habitually come unprepared should be sent off the unit, and the day should be counted as an unexcused absence. Check the school policy covering this situation.

Another part of validating preparation is assessing if the student is physically and mentally ready to care for patients. Some students stay up so late working on their care plans that they are not fit to implement them. Decide whether it would be better to send the student home with some words to the wise for better planning in the future. The reason for the student's situation will determine whether to count this as an excused or unexcused absence.

Other students may have their functioning altered in other ways, such as by drugs or alcohol. It is unfortunate that this must be mentioned, but it happens. These students should always be sent home. Be certain that the specific behavior is documented. Ask the student to account for the questionable behavior and discuss the situation with the course coordinator.

Clarifying Student Roles

It is often difficult to get across to beginning students what they can and cannot do. Some beginning students have done more as nurse techs than they are initially allowed to do as nursing students. They need some help in understanding the role transition. Other students may focus so much on the limits that they cannot see how much latitude they do have. Emphasize to them that they should be conservative and that if they are in doubt, they should ask questions. When they are about to make assumptions, the newer they are, the more they need to check their assumptions.

Being a Participant Observer

Acute Care Settings

In medical-surgical settings, faculty are likely to be involved in helping students provide care, especially with newer students. Faculty members doing this should be aware that they are serving as role models. In addition, observe the students' behavior in order to evaluate progress or to identify learning needs.

Develop a comfortable style that will enable observation without disturbing the student. Smile and greet both the student and patient when you enter the room. Exchanging a little friendly banter helps to dispel the anxiety the student may feel about being observed.

Participate in the patient's care in a way that feels natural to the patient. For example, if a student seems to be having trouble figuring out how to remove the patient's gown when the patient is connected to an IV, say something like, "That is a tough one. Let me show you how I do it." This conveys to the student that this is just one of those things it takes time to learn, and it keeps the patient from having to worry about what the student is doing.

If the student is about to do something unsafe, such as contaminate a sterile field or administer an injection in the wrong site, try to be as unobtrusive as possible about drawing the student's attention to it. Stop the student verbally if necessary and try to manage the situation in such a way that the student does not look or feel incompetent. For example, with a student who is catheterizing a patient and about to contaminate the tip of the catheter, calmly say, "Try holding the catheter closer to the tip. Those things wiggle a lot if you hold them too far down the tubing." This is much less distracting than engaging at this time in questions and answers about sterile fields or the physical characteristics of urinary catheters.

When students make errors, talk to them privately as soon as possible about what happened. Encourage the student to analyze what went wrong and to figure out the reasons for it. Discuss ways to prevent errors from occurring again. Let students know that they should feel comfortable asking questions when in doubt.

Even with patience and guidance, some students cannot see that they did anything wrong, or they cannot think of a correct alternative. Tell these students directly what was wrong and what they should have done. Such students need close supervision.

Ambulatory Care Settings

It is sometimes harder to observe students in clinics than in hospital units because it is harder to keep track of where they are. It helps to have a central location where students can leave a note on a clipboard as to which examination room they are in or where they have gone if they have left the clinic.

When and how students are supervised in clinic settings depends on the purpose of the students' being there. If the experience is strictly observational, the students need guidelines for their behavior. For example, they need to know what to say if anyone asks them to demonstrate a skill. The best response to such a request would be for the student to say that he or she cannot help but will go and get someone who has the needed expertise.

Students need some guidance in knowing what they are to observe. For example, the focus may be on the roles of the nurse in the clinic or may be on the identification of nursing interventions that would be helpful to the clinic clients.

If students are expected to demonstrate skills and assist nurses or physicians, the acceptable skills should be specified. The nurses and physicians in the clinic need to know the limitations on student activities. In order to observe a student, arrange to be present at the initiation of an examination or procedure. This will be less distracting to the student, other health care workers, and the client than entering a room during some activity would be.

Home Visits

It is difficult to be unobtrusive when the patient, the student, and the faculty are sitting in the patient's living room. In the first place, having the student there is an unusual event in the patient's life. At the beginning of the visit, the faculty member should clarify the reason for student's being there. Some patients will tend to talk to the faculty when they should be talking to the student. Redirect the communication to the student. Find out in advance what the student plans to say to the patient. Help the student to fill in gaps or correct misconceptions before the visit.

Fostering a Positive Climate for Learning

Expectations

One thing that helps to make students feel safe and comfortable in a learning situation is knowledge of what is expected of them. Try to give students an idea of what observations faculty will be making in the clinical setting. When discussing performance, link comments to specific objectives and course requirements.

There are some aspects of expected clinical behavior for students that faculty assume the students know, but the students' actions show they do not. For example, in one case, a student in a community health setting was working with a patient whose son would start crying as soon as he saw anyone in uniform. After this happened the first time that the student went to visit the family, the student was given permission to visit the family wearing street clothes. The faculty assumed that the student knew this was an exception for that one situation. The student assumed that because it would be complicated to change clothes before or after the visits, she could wear street clothes on all her visits. When the student and one of the staff nurses made a visit together to another family, the staff nurse confronted her about her inappropriate attire. The student told her that the faculty member had approved it, so the nurse approached the faculty, and the confusion was rectified.

Assertiveness

One of the expectations for students is for them to become assertive and to take initiative in giving nursing care. Be sure the students understand the limits their initiative can take. When students are assertive, reinforce this behavior. For example, Dan was assigned to a patient whose left leg was in a full leg cast. The woman was in her 50s and had been to physical therapy earlier in the morning. She had not been back on the unit for long before she was scheduled to walk with crutches on the unit. She told the student that she was too tired from physical therapy and wanted to rest for a while before trying crutch-walking. When the nurse asked Dan why he did not get the patient up on crutches, he told her what the patient had said. The nurse told him the patient was lazy. Dan pointed out to the nurse that the woman was not accustomed to much physical exertion, she had only been up on crutches once before, and she had had an extensive session in physical therapy. He said he would not label the patient as lazy, and he thought it was legitimate for her to wait until later in the morning for more activity.

Even when students make mistakes, try to foster assertiveness while helping them examine and correct the behavior.

Self-Esteem

Whenever one is in a student role, self-esteem is greatly affected by one's learning experiences. In teaching nursing, many of the young people have been students for virtually their entire lives. Their self-concepts tend to center around being students, and things that happen to them in this role determine their self-esteem. This helps to explain why they can get so passionate about the difference between an A and a B on a test, for example.

In the clinical area, students have their behavior evaluated in a way that most of them have never experienced in another situation. This is a much more emotionally laden experience than is marking answers on a test or writing a term paper. A lot of what students are evaluated on may relate to their personalities. For example, the way a student interacts with a patient is partially determined by that student's culture, family, personal experiences, and self-concept. When a faculty member critiques the student's skill, deeply held beliefs and values may be threatened, however unintentionally. Because of this, a student's reactions to the faculty member's remarks may sometimes be perplexing.

An insecure student may treat a comment that was meant to be just a suggestion as a mandate. Another comment intended to be funny may hurt a student's feelings. The problem is that faculty probably will not realize immediately that such comments have had these results.

When students make mistakes, do not heap blame or criticism on them. They are often much harder on themselves than necessary. Be sure that students appreciate the impact of errors they make, but also help them to put such incidents in perspective. Students need to know when they are doing well. Let them know this as directly as possible. Rather than simply saying, "You met the objectives," add specific positive comments, such as, "You were so gentle, and it was obvious the patient appreciated it," or "You did that as if you had been doing it all your life," or "Yes, it was a little prolonged, but you explained everything so well that I do not think it bothered the patient."

The clinical faculty member is the expert whose role is to make judgments about each student's performance. Part of making those judgments is helping students to reinforce strengths, not just to eliminate weaknesses. Students should end their experience knowing more about nursing but also feeling more confident about themselves as they evolve into professional nurses.

Describe behavior and explain why it is or is not acceptable. Avoid putting global labels on students or their behavior. For example, do not say, "You are incompetent." Describe what is wrong and why it is a problem. Please do not ever say, "You are never going to be a good nurse," or words to that effect. In the first place, the faculty could be wrong. Maybe that student will be a fantastic nurse in a different setting. In the second place, such a statement does not offer any room for growth.

Faculty members sometimes get very upset with students or undermine students' self-esteem, particularly when situations arise that may reflect on the clinical ability of faculty.

A faculty member who worries about being blamed may get defensive and show it by getting angry with the student. This faculty member could also get depressed and not look at how the incident could be used to improve student orientation. Faculty should know that they are not perfect and students are not perfect. As long as we are also trying to do all we can to promote safe care, the chances of those mistakes being serious are limited.

Helping Students in Difficulty

Overidentification

Sometimes students have trouble with patients when they overidentify with the patient or the patient's situation. This often shows up when the student manifests an extreme behavior such as (1) spending too much time or not enough time with the patient, (2) being too restrictive or too permissive with the patient's behavior, (3) arguing with others about the care the patient is or is not getting, (4) doing too much or too little for the patient, or (5) seeming too confident or too reticent in dealing with the patient.

When signals like these are observed, make it a point to talk with the student. Although the student may start out being defensive, he or she may be able to volunteer the information that helps to explain what is happening. For example, a student working with an alcoholic who reminds her of her father may behave inappropriately. With help, she will be able to begin separating her feelings and responsibilities about one individual from those about the other.

It is obviously more difficult to work with a student who denies the overidentification. Continue to point out behaviors that are inappropriate and try to help the student see this more objectively. However, the student will have trouble attaining objectivity while still working with the patient. If the student's problem interferes with what is in the patient's best interest, change the student's assignment.

Blocking

Sometimes a student freezes when it is time to do a new procedure, especially if it is an invasive one. It is fairly common for students to have some anxiety about giving their first injections. A few will become immobilized by the anxiety. One of my students gave me no clues that she was any more nervous than the average student about giving her first injection to a patient. We entered the room, she told the patient what she was there for, and she positioned him properly for an injection in his buttock. She pointed out the correct site to me, swabbed it with alcohol, and removed the cap from the needle. My attention was directed to the man's hip, and I realized that nothing else seemed to be happening. I looked back at her to see a wide, unblinking stare. I patted her shoulder and nodded for her to go on, as I pointed at the site and smiled encouragingly. Nothing happened. I gently extracted the syringe from her hand and gave the injection myself. She swabbed the man's skin and rearranged the covers over him. I made sure he was comfortable, and we left the room. She leaned against the wall and looked like she might faint or start crying, so I ushered her into an empty room. We talked about what had happened, and I assured her I understood her behavior. She finally said that she wanted another chance as soon as possible. One of the staff nurses was about to get an injection for one of her patients, and she let the student draw it up. This time, when we went to the room, the student did fine

Sometimes when students block on giving injections or on some other procedure, they almost have an anxiety attack about it. It is best not to push them too hard because this extreme blocking represents a severe form of anxiety. Try to work around that particular skill for a while.

Another kind of student blocking happens when you enter the room to observe. No matter how unthreatening, faculty will probably make students nervous when watching the students' performance. It is part of the nature of the situation. Some of this anxiety diminishes as the students have experiences in which faculty are helpful and supportive to them.

However, some students have a chronic problem with this. Try to arrange to do things with them rather than just stand and observe them. Arrange to talk with the student before an observation and be clear about the purpose.

Fortunately, most students get over blocking anxiety, or they learn to function well, even though they are still nervous. If they cannot overcome the anxiety or learn to function, and if it is just one student here or there, the faculty is not likely to be the real cause. In severe situations, the students may need outside counseling. Talk to the course coordinator before referring students for counseling on such matters.

If many students seem to become very anxious when observed or block when they are trying to perform, the faculty should reflect on their own behaviors. Be objective. Ask a colleague to observe and help identify what may be causing these reactions. Without intending to give such an impression, faculty may seem very stern and unfriendly, causing even secure students to become disorganized.

Conflicts

If a student has a conflict with a patient, try to figure out what is going on so that, unless the patient demands that the student not continue, the student can keep working with the patient. As with most conflicts, sometimes it is the patient's problem, sometimes it is the student's problem, and sometimes it is a combination. Sometimes students are slow in doing things. Although some patients accept this, others are not able to tolerate it. Slow students usually need more practice or more support to learn to function faster. However, some patients may be very distressed by this behavior.

If students get into conflicts with staff, assess why this is happening. First, find out both sides of the story by talking with the staff members involved and with the student. Get specific descriptions of behaviors related to the conflict. Try to avoid a direct confrontation between staff and student.

Sometimes, a student will be abrasive. Preserve the learning experience for the student and be supportive of the staff. They make it possible for all students to learn. If the student is in the wrong, help the student understand what is wrong, but also assure the staff you have intervened, without unduly embarrassing the student.

Serious conflicts between staff and students are rare. When it does happen, it is sometimes because of a particular staff member who has a history of problems with many students and who openly objects to working with nursing students. Other conflicts occur because of a problem the student is having. For example, some students are judgmental and condescending to the staff. Other students are poorly organized or overly dependent. These students will bother the staff. When confronted, the student is likely to blame the staff rather than accept responsibility.

Finally, sometimes faculty will have conflicts with students. Conflict usually arises because of differing expectations. If the conflict seems to be with only one or two students, it is most likely an issue related to these students as individuals and not a larger problem with the faculty member. Have the same expectations of all students and apply grading criteria equitably. Some new faculty members expect too much from their students, for example. Others are so concerned about the welfare of the patients that this is conveyed to the students as a lack of trust in them.

Knowing More Than the Students

Sometimes your students will ask questions you cannot answer. Do not try to fake it. Give them the message that it is okay to still be learning even when you are a professional.

Do not try to evade a question by merely sending a student off to "look it up." Suggest that the student and faculty find out the answer together.

This shows the student that learning is ongoing. Helping a student to identify sources of knowledge is an important aspect of clinical experiences. Students need to know what they do not know and more importantly need to know where to find the information.

Anecdotal Notes

Most faculty members keep a record of the important aspects of students' performance through anecdotal notes. As the name implies, the notes report anecdotal comments about the students' progress in the clinical area. Such notes help in day-to-day counseling of students and provide data for evaluation. Make note of accomplishments as well as of learning needs indicated by incidents in the clinical area.

Form

The form is probably the least important aspect of anecdotal records. You can use a PDA, a notebook, or whatever is convenient. Entries are usually fairly explicit and document incidents that support how the student is or is not meeting the objectives.

Timeliness

The most important requirement is that this record be made as close as possible in time to the actual events. It is easy to forget and distort things with the passage of time, so it helps to write down comments as soon as possible.

Content

The content should be made up of descriptive observations about the students' behavior. This will help in writing evaluations and can better help the students to understand how conclusions were drawn. Avoid judgmental statements. Table 2.1 shows a sample anecdotal note.

TABLE 2.1   Anecdotal Note

Note on Leah   9/19/05
Worked w/32 y/o woman, postop 2 days, splenectomy. L. asked pt. when she wanted bath and planned around it. Found out woman was trying to lose weight and wanted a diet. L. got order for this & informed dietary. Planned for this, keeping in mind need for her body to heal. Did not check chart for new orders & was late giving 1st dose of new med. I would not have known this, but she told me herself, as well as how she would avoid this oversight in future.

Access

Anecdotal notes should be treated as confidential documents. Although these notes are confidential, the course coordinator or grievance board could request them if there is any question about the student evaluation and final grade.

Evaluating Clinical Performance

Clinical Content

The specifics of what students should accomplish in the clinical area are determined by the objectives. The particular clinical area as well as school policy will determine the way students are evaluated. Some programs have very specific expectations with levels of achievement identified, so that number or letter grades can be given. Other programs may have certain minimum expectations that all students must achieve, but the grade for clinical is "Satisfactory" or "Unsatisfactory."

The clearer the expectations and their association with the grading system, the less difficult it is to arrive at a grade. There is no way to avoid the fact that evaluating clinical performance is subjective. Objectively written criteria minimize subjectivity. However, even the application of objective criteria is affected by the values of the person assessing the performance. For example, two faculty members might both observe a skill exercised by a student. One might be more flexible about deviations from the usual way this is done as long as the student does it safely and ends up with the correct result. The other might think it is important to include every step just as he or she learned it in the first place. On the other hand, the stricter faculty member might allow students to be more casual in their interactions with patients than the other expects. These differences could lead to different grades. However, the more explicit the criteria and the more agreement there is about expectations and values, the closer the two faculty members will be in assigning grades.

With experience, you will become more confident. Develop a grading rubric for each assignment will help faculty give similar grades. Share the grading rubric with students so that the process is transparent.

In some clinical settings, it may be useful to develop a learning contract. This helps to make expectations explicit and makes it clearer that the students determine their grades by their behavior. Chapter 3 describes that process of developing such a contract.

TABLE 2.2 Behaviors Implying the Presence of Professional Values

Value: Placing the patient's welfare first
Is accessible and prompt in answering patients' requests
Priority of activities reflects patients' needs
Explains treatments and procedures; keeps patient well informed Is responsive and reliable when needs are identified by patients, staff, or faculty
Calls and makes appropriate arrangements if unable to be on time or present for clinical

Value: Commitment to nursing and to nursing department policies
Present and willing to learn; complies voluntarily with rules and policies of the nursing department
Demonstrates enthusiasm for clinical; appears to enjoy nursing
Looks and acts in a professional manner (i.e., is neat and clean; behaves in a professional way)
Pleasant to staff, peers, and faculty
Gives appropriate information to other nurses
Completes charts and records

Value: Cooperation
Able to disagree diplomatically
Knows when to stop arguing and start helping
Takes criticism constructively
Accepts the roles of others and works in appropriate capacity in response to others
Deals with stress and frustration without taking it out on others
Objectively handles conflict with others; tries to see both sides of issues

Value: Intellectual and personal integrity
Readily admits mistakes and oversights
Forthright with peers, staff, and faculty
Selects appropriate response to patients even if preferring to focus on something else
Observes safe techniques even when not being supervised
Accepts responsibility for errors and tries to take appropriate corrective action
Statements appear to be based on fact and believable; does not provide information or facts unless known to be correct
Does own work and does not represent the work of others as being original
Respectful of faculty, staff, peers, and patients

Professional Behavior

Unlike some content-related behaviors, there are certain professional expectations that are either present or absent. Sometimes it may be difficult to spell out these expectations, which are as significant as any expectations

TABLE 2.3   Behaviors Implying the Absence of Professional Values

Value: Placing the patient's welfare first
Unreliable in completion of tasks
Difficult to find when needed
Elicits hostility from patients and others
Displays hostility toward difficult patients
Justifies doing things "just for the experience," without taking patients' needs into consideration
Approach is "who is right," not "what is right"
Fails to make appropriate arrangements if unable to be on time or present for clinical

Value: Commitment to nursing and to nursing department policies
Chronically tardy or absent
Skips clinical or other obligations if not supervised
Passes off assignments or tasks to others when possible
Chronic malcontent and complainer
Sloppy
Gives inappropriate information to others
Chronically deficient in upkeep of charts and records
Feels existent policies are irrelevant, unimportant, and nonobligatory

Value: Cooperation
Argumentative or stubborn
Sullen or arrogant with faculty, peers, staff, and patients
Uncommunicative with staff and faculty
Hostile responses to frustrating situations
Passive-aggressive behavior when dissatisfied

Value: Intellectual and personal integrity
Lies or fabricates data to cover up mistakes and oversights
Fails to use safe techniques when not being supervised
Blames others for own shortcomings
Provides data without appropriate checks for correctness
Sneaks away or does not show up if unsupervised
Represents the work of others as being original
Disrespectful and rude to faculty, staff, peers, or patients

related to safe patient care. Tables 2.2 and 2.3 show lists of behaviors that indicate the presence or absence of values related to professionalism.

Frequently, the most concerning area with students relates to their inability to provide nursing care in a professional way. Even though they make good grades, they seem to lack a real concern or regard for patients. It is legitimate to build these expectations into grading criteria. Specifying such expectations and spelling out that students must consistently demonstrate these behaviors gives support if these behaviors must be adhered to in order to pass clinical.

Formative and Summative

Formative evaluation is the process that helps a student to achieve the final objectives. Usually this evaluation is informal, such as telling students on a weekly basis how they have done in the clinical area. At the midpoint of the term, give a slightly more formal evaluation of students' performance so that they know what they have accomplished and what they need to achieve in the remainder of the term. Generally, a grade is not attached to such assessments because they are meant to promote growth. Summative evaluations are the evaluations that are done at the end of an experience in order to evaluate the students' ability to meet the terminal objectives. A grade is usually attached to summative evaluations.

Evaluating students on a day-to-day basis is a formative process. Although the clinical practice time may be compressed, students need to be allowed to practice skills and behaviors before they are actually graded on them. Students become intimidated when faculty begin grading behaviors immediately. How can they feel they are really in a learning environment if they are penalized for needing to learn?

Conferences

Preclinical

Some faculty members have a brief conference with students at the beginning of the clinical day in order to share information, validate preparation, or simply convey information. This is usually fairly short, especially if it is prior to the day shift.

Postclinical

It is very common for faculty to meet in conference with students after their daily or weekly clinical experience. Determine what will be covered in these conferences, which may include, for example, conveying content, such as explicit details of a procedure, or discussing the salient events the students experienced during the clinical period.

Some faculty members expect students to take turns in presenting their patients to the rest of the group. The focus can be on the use of the nursing process or on a specific problem. The conference could be used to review specific activities or objectives and to review how the students accomplished these.

This is also a good opportunity for vicarious learning, such as when a student has had a unique experience to share with the group. Nurse managers or other clinical personnel can be invited to come for a specific purpose.

FINAL WORDS

Supervising students in any clinical area may produce high degrees of anxiety for students and faculty. As faculty gain experience, they become less anxious. Try to make it as positive and growth-producing as possible for the student.

FURTHER READING

Adams, V. (2002). Consistent clinical assignment for nursing students compared to multiple placements. *Journal of Nursing Education, 41*(2), 80.

Murphy, J. (2004). Using focused reflection and articulation to promote clinical reassuring: An evidenced based teaching strategy. *Nursing Education Perspectives, 25*(5), 226–236.

3

Designing a Learning Contract

A learning contract is one method of planning students' work and determining students' success. The learning contract places the responsibility for and control of the learning in the hands of the student. The faculty member begins by specifying the amount and quality of work required for each grade. Then the student chooses the grades for which they are willing to work. This is helpful in courses with requirements that make grading difficult as well as in those that have several clinical sections graded by different instructors. For example, some assignments may be easier to evaluate in terms of the degree of students' participation if the quality of the participation is not easily assessed. A study of a community agency may yield the same basic data for a good or a weak student. However, students have the opportunity to receive higher grades by investing more time in the study, by interviewing a wider variety of staff or clients, or by spending more time in the agency.

Contract grading makes it clear that the performance of the student is directly connected to the grade. Students can choose how much effort they are willing to put into a given course or assignment. This method is often used with clinical grading, but it is also useful with other complex assignments. The option of choosing how much effort to expend gives the students more autonomy in meeting the goals of clinical practice or an assignment.

One of the advantages of using contracts is that students feel less competition with each another. If they all contract for an A and achieve all the work necessary, they can all earn an A. Contracts make expectations explicit, so students feel there is more objectivity on the part of faculty. A disadvantage frequently cited by faculty and students is that contracts seem to place more emphasis on quantity than on quality. However, building in qualitative criteria along with other contract elements rectifies this.

GOALS

The principal goal of using contracts in evaluating and grading students is to increase student autonomy. Contract grading also promotes objectivity in evaluation.

TOOLS

Objectives

The objectives for the clinical experience or assignment determine the format for the contract. Regardless of the grade for which the student contracts, each student has to meet every objective to some extent. The contract specifies how that must be done for each grade.

Format

Table 3.1 outlines the principal components of the contract material. The example is from the clinical component of a course in community health nursing.

Introduction

Start with an introduction that explains the use of the contract. This will be a new experience for many students. They need a general idea of what will be involved.

Objectives

List the objectives that students will meet by following the contract. It is important for students to see that there are connections between contract specifications and the objectives.

Performance Requirements

List the performance requirements for each grade level. Usually, all students are supposed to meet the basic performance standards. As they work to achieve higher grades, additional work may be expected for each increment. In addition, students working toward higher grades may be expected to meet higher qualitative standards of practice when they complete the basic requirements.

TABLE 3.1 Contract Requirements for Community Health Clinical Experience

Introduction: The purpose of the contract is to permit you (the student) to determine the amount and quality of work for the clinical experience. After reading the requirements for each grade, complete the contract form and be prepared to discuss it with your instructor at the set time.

Objectives: At the end of this clinical experience, you will be able to do the following:

1. Plan and carry out home visits to clients in their homes.
2. Describe and analyze interpersonal interactions with clients.
3. Develop and maintain ongoing nursing care plans for clients in the community.
4. Plan and implement effective teaching strategies with community clients.
5. Make appropriate referrals for community clients.
6. Describe and compare the roles of nurses in the community.

Performance Requirements:

Grade of C

1. Follow one client or family, and perform the following tasks:

    (a) Make weekly home visits.

    (b) Maintain appropriate records at the agency.

    (c) Maintain an ongoing nursing care plan.

    (d) Have written objectives for each visit.

    (e) Maintain drug cards as needed.

    (f) Make appropriate referrals as needed.

2. Submit your care plan to the instructor each week.
3. Meet with the instructor weekly to discuss the progress of work with your client.
4. Attend and participate in weekly group conference with instructor and peers.
5. Attend clinics and other activities as scheduled once a week.
6. Complete one process recording that meets minimum requirements as specified in course syllabus.
7. Complete one teaching project that meets minimum requirements.
8. Using contract criteria, complete weekly self-evaluations and a summative evaluation at the end of the term.

Grade of B

1. Meet all the requirements for a grade of C; in addition, the nursing care plan, teaching plan, and process recording must meet B-level criteria as specified in the course syllabus.

(continued)

TABLE 3.1 *(Continued)*

2. Follow one additional client or family, meeting the same expectations as with the first client or family.

3. Read three journal articles on the clinical application of community theory and prepare bibliography cards on the articles.

Grade of A

1. Meet all the requirements for a grade of C; in addition, the nursing care plan, teaching plan, and process recording must meet A-level criteria as specified in the course syllabus.

2. Follow one additional client or family meeting the same expectations as with the first client or family.

3. Read three journal articles on the clinical application of community theory and prepare bibliography cards on the articles.

4. Complete a special-focus process recording (PR) with specific learning objectives agreed upon with the clinical instructor. The PR must reflect creativity and meet the criteria for the A level.

5. Write a brief paper (three to four typed pages) focusing on the counseling role of the nurse; use at least two references and include one or more examples from your own clinical experience.

Contract Form

The final component is the actual contract to be signed by each student and the instructor, specifying the intended grade. The contract form should include a section for reviewing and renegotiating at a given point. Table 3.2 shows a contract form to go with the material in Table 3.1.

Checklist

Another item that may be helpful is a checklist to initial as a student satisfies each requirement. Space can be incorporated for evaluative comments. At the end of the term, this checklist provides the basis for the evaluation, and a copy can be filed in lieu of some other form. An example checklist is shown in Table 3.3.

NUTS AND BOLTS

Deadlines

Set deadlines for each activity. Students who want extensions may negotiate for new deadlines.

TABLE 3.2 Contract Form

Community Health Clinical Student Contract

This form is to be signed by you (the student) and the faculty member by the end of the first clinical week. After reading the performance requirements, you will indicate the grade you will work toward. If you do not satisfy all the requirements for the contracted grade, you will receive the grade for which you have met requirements.

At any time during the term, you may ask to renegotiate. If you want to change to a higher grade, sufficient time must remain for you to achieve that grade. If you want to change to a lower grade, any commitments to clients must be completed.

I, _____ , have read the performance requirements for the community health clinical experience and will work for a grade of ___.

_____   _____

Student   Clinical instructor

I wish to change the original terms. As of this date, I will work for a grade of ___.

_____   _____

Student   Clinical instructor

Validation

The student should carry the primary responsibility in asking faculty to validate that contract requirements have been met. This is especially important in acute care settings where many of the requirements may involve psychomotor skills.

When students are ready to demonstrate competence with a required skill, they should find the instructor and request supervision for this purpose. The student should carry a copy of the checklist so that there are no problems later with transferring needed information.

In other settings, the checklist affords a good guide to help the students stay on top of their responsibilities. Even while using the checklist, make anecdotal notes to support decisions about the quality of the student's performance.

Criteria

Specify the criteria used to give different letter grades for certain assignments. This is important because it helps to demonstrate that achieving

TABLE 3.3   Contract Checklist

Student_____ Term_____

Contracted grade____

Criteria for all clinical activities will be at the level described in the course syllabus as determined by the contracted grade.

Requirements for all grades:

1. Client/family visits

Weeks	1	2	3	4
Visited weekly				
Record entries				
Care plan in				
Objectives				
Drug cards				
Referrals				

2. Meet with instructor
3. Group conferences
4. Clinics
5. PR turned in
6. Teaching project
7. Self-evaluations

Additional requirements for B and A:

1. Second client/family

Weeks	1	2	3	4
Visited weekly				
Record entries				
Care plan in				
Objectives				
Drug cards				
Referrals				

2. Bibliography cards   No. 1   No. 2   No. 3

Additional requirements for A:

1. Special PR
2. Clinical paper

Comments:

higher grades according to the contract is not dependent only on quantity. Table 3.4 shows some criteria that could be used to differentiate among the levels when evaluating a teaching plan.

For some activities, you may simply require the student to complete the work, but not evaluate the work using the criteria. An example would be the observations made in clinics as part of the community health clinical activities.

Giving a Numerical Grade

With most assignments, use a numerical grade as well as a letter grade so that this can be averaged with other components of a course grade. This is the point at which subjectivity is bound to enter. A student may consistently meet the expectations for the contracted letter grade and perhaps even do as well as the next-higher letter on some things. Give the student the highest number in the range for the letter grade.

Another student may barely meet the qualitative criteria and may take a long time to start demonstrating skills consistently at the contracted grade level. That student might receive a lower number in the grade's range. One thing to remember is that a grade of 100 for an A does not mean the student is perfect. It merely means that the student consistently accomplished the requirements set for an A for that course.

If students receive a letter grade for the clinical portion of the course, no matter what the means of reaching the grade, some students will try to manipulate faculty into giving them a few more points. This is especially true if a few points may raise their course grades to a higher letter. Suddenly, someone who could not find the time to look up one extra reference for a teaching plan will invest an hour in trying to get two more points for the clinical grade. (See Table 3.4.)

Using the Contract

Many students determine for themselves that they do not want to do the work required for a grade of A. Some students have objected to the contract, feeling they might have received higher grades if the requirements had not been so specific.

TABLE 3.4 Grade-Level Criteria for Teaching Plan[a]

C Level	B Level	A Level
Assessment		
Obvious data identified	Obvious & subtle data identified	Obvious & subtle data identified
Uses readily available references	Uses additional references	Uses additional references
Nursing dx is obvious	Nursing dx is obvious	Nursing dx is subtle
Planning		
States obvious behavioral obj. that can be measured	All obvious behavioral obj. are stated clearly & are measurable	All obvious & some subtle obj. are stated clearly & are measurable
Implementation		
Obvious teaching methods with limited skill & preparation used correctly	Teaching methods with moderate preparation & limited skill used correctly	Teaching methods with extensive preparation & moderate skill used correctly
Obvious content is identified	All applicable content is identified	All applicable content is identified
Rationale for methods & content are described & documented by assigned texts	Rationale for methods & content are described & documented by 1 or 2 resources in addition to texts	Rationale for methods & content are described & documented by more than 2 resources in addition to texts
Evaluation		
Methods & content are evaluated	Methods & content are evaluated as to effectiveness & appropriateness	Methods & content are evaluated as to effectiveness & appropriateness with discussion of future use
Client's ability to meet each behavioral objective is described	Client's ability to meet each behavioral objective is described	Client's ability to meet each behavioral objective is evaluated in a creative way

[a] Adapted from Schoolcraft & Delaney (1982).

On the other hand, try to talk students into trying for higher grades when they do not feel confident in themselves. After a few days in clinical, if the student is doing a lot better than the contracted grade requires, encourage that student to consider doing the additional work. This builds self-confidence and a positive learning outcome.

Try to give students as much time as reasonable to accomplish the grades they choose. For example, a student contracting for an A may be a slow starter. Give the student as much time as possible to get in the groove. If it becomes apparent that the student cannot handle the expectations, suggest developing a contract for a lower grade.

FINAL WORDS

Learning contracts offer a way to give the student more independence in the clinical area. Contracts help to defuse some of the anxiety that students experience when the instructor observes them because the students can determine when they are ready to be evaluated. They know in advance which criteria they have to meet. The contract option does not remove all the difficulties of grading, but it can help a lot.

FURTHER READING

Chan, S. W., & Wai-tong, C. (2000). Implementing contract learning in a clinical context. *Journal of Advanced Nursing, 31*(2), 298–305.

4

Teaching Students to Work in Groups

Nurses and other health care providers work in teams. Therefore, it makes sense that faculty require nursing students to accomplish certain assignments by working together. We need reasonable expectations of students so that we do not ask too much of them when we give these assignments. If expectations are not appropriate for the students, students may become so bogged down in the group process that they are unable to learn what is expected in terms of content.

Although some faculty members give students guidance in working together, many do not. Some faculty members may expect everyone to be familiar with this aspect of teamwork without thinking about where anyone is supposed to acquire the necessary skills. Frequently, faculty members consider group dynamics to be only in the purview of psychiatric and mental health faculty. By the time students get to their mental health courses, they already may have worked on group assignments and may have learned some poor habits if the faculty who covered group dynamics intentionally or unintentionally linked the theory only with group therapy rather than with more general applications. If students have not been exposed to concepts about effective group work, plan to teach this skill.

GOALS

The primary goal of teaching the dynamics of group functioning is to promote effective group work. A secondary goal is to foster student appreciation of the use of groups in working on problems.

TOOLS

Guidelines for Effective Group Work

Structure

Set some of the structural aspects, such as the number of students who will work in each group, how the group membership will be determined, and the focus of their work together. Three or four students would be an optimal number. If part of the purpose of having students work together is to focus on group process, more than two in a group is necessary. If more than five students are in a group, the workload may be spread too thin, or some students may not participate equitably.

Assign students to the group membership, or allow students to select their own partners. If the group work is going to take several hours out of class, let students pick their own partners to make it easier for them to arrange group meetings. If the group work is to take place during class time, assign people to groups in order to help them to get to know and work with people other than their friends.

Establish the focus when you describe the assignment and set the objectives. Students may focus on both content and process, in which case you should set objectives for both. For example, in a community course taught by one of the authors of this book, some of the objectives focused on the students' group process. A written paper addressed the content of the study. The students also dealt with their process by submitting a written statement about their respective responsibilities; discussing their work together when they met with the faculty member; and writing a summary of their group work that was submitted with the final paper.

Other structural aspects have to be worked out by each group. Provide them with some guidance in doing this. A timetable such as the one in Table 4.1 may help the students to accomplish their work. They could use this timetable as it is or could develop a more detailed one that specifies the agenda for each meeting.

Process

In addition to specifying the expectations for their performance in the group, give the students some help in working together. Giving them printed guidelines or ground rules is helpful, especially when engaging

TABLE 4.1   Timetable for Group Work

First Meeting

1. Identify focus (e.g., assignment or problem).
2. Discuss approach and distribute work.

   Assign individual responsibilities.

   Determine group responsibilities.
3. Establish a schedule and deadlines.
4. Plan for presentation of report.

   (a) Oral: Set time to assign parts and plan format.

   (b) Written: Arrange for typing, proofing, and submitting document.

Other Meetings

1. Review work done by individuals.
2. Do group work.
3. Assess progress in meeting deadlines.
4. Identify problems and work on solutions.

Last Meeting

1. Assemble individual work and review as a group.
2. Complete group work.
3. Make final arrangements for presentation of report.

them in a simulation to practice these behaviors. Table 4.2 lists some guidelines for consideration.

Simulations

A simulation is a structured experience allowing students the opportunity to practice skills prior to using them in real-world situations. Simulations may be used to help students learn group skills in general, or they may help students to practice before undertaking a specific group project. Simulations of problem-solving and creative-thinking situations and other kinds of group exercises can be helpful in conveying useful theory as well

TABLE 4.2   Effective and Creative Group Work

Promoting Effective Thinking

1. Make expectations explicit.
2. Take risks and persevere.
3. Expand perceptions.
4. Challenge assumptions.
5. Suspend judgment.
6. Foster self-esteem.
7. Be patient.
8. Tolerate ambiguity and chaos.

Fostering a Supportive Group

1. All the group members should have the right to protect their self-image.
2. Aggression in the group should be directed toward the problem, not toward group members.
3. Effective group work results in everyone winning.

Brainstorming Ground Rules

1. No criticism of ideas should be allowed during the brainstorming phase.
2. "Far out" ideas are encouraged because they may trigger other, more practical ideas from someone else.
3. Quantity of ideas is more important than quality.

as in providing an opportunity for application. For example, the following question could be considered for each small group, using the guidelines in Table 4.2: "How can you find out, in an unobtrusive way, what the people in a given community see as their highest health concern?"

NUTS AND BOLTS

Supervision of Group Assignments

Build in some ongoing contact with groups as they work through a complex assignment. If students are having trouble with either the content or the group process, faculty can help them before they get completely lost. With undergraduates it is a good idea to set up specific meeting times.

If some group members are not doing their share, the other members may be taking on extra work rather than dealing with an unpleasant confrontation. Faculty members fail to deal with such problems within their own ranks, yet they penalize students for not handling these incidents directly.

Try to help students identify their own problems. If they cannot, point out the problems. Set limits and talk to students who are not pulling their own weight. A lower grade may be warranted. The example situation described next illustrates the complexities of dealing with a problem student.

One student did not show up for the planned meetings with the rest of the group. When other members of the group brought this up in a meeting, the student in question began to give excuses about why she did not come and why she did not contact the others. They reported reasonable efforts to contact her, including trying to talk to her in class. When any of them approached her, she always had a reason for not being able to talk. The faculty member told her that if she did not figure out some way to meet with the group and do her share of the work, she would receive a failing grade for the assignment. She got angry and insisted on being allowed to do the assignment herself. The student was told that it was meant as a group assignment, and it seemed unlikely that she could manage it on her own. She finally agreed to work on the part she had originally been assigned. When the group submitted their paper, the faculty member met with them and asked each student in turn to describe what she or he did. The one who had the problems with participating had clearly done less than the others, had given her part to the others late, and had not read the rest of the paper. She did not earn the same grade as the others and was given a grade based only on the quality of her work.

Using Simulations

The criteria for selecting simulations or exercises should relate to the learning goals for students as well as to faculty level of expertise in facilitating group work.

Criteria:

- The exercise achieves the identified goals.
- The exercise fits with earlier and later exercises.
- Materials required can be easily obtained or are easy to construct.
- Facilitation of the exercise can be clearly described in written steps.
- The exercise is not likely to be emotionally distressing to the participants.
- The exercise is interesting and fun to do.
- The exercise is easy to facilitate.

These criteria can help faculty members who have little background in facilitating groups.

Designing an Exercise

Start by writing out the steps in the exercise. Try it out on a group of your colleagues or friends before trying it with students. This will establish some important factors: the actual time involved, the clarity of the instructions, and the suitability to accomplish the goals.

There are many concepts that can be demonstrated to students by using group activities. As a matter of fact, using an experiential approach often has a great deal more impact than simply telling about the concept. Some exercises to consider are the following:

- Group-task and group-maintenance roles assumed by group members
- Thinking creatively
- Group problem-solving
- Effect of synergy in group problem-solving
- Benefits of two-way communication as contrasted with one-way communication
- Distortions that occur when rumors are spread
- Assertive behavior
- Effective group planning
- Outcomes of competition and cooperation

See Table 4.3.

TABLE 4.3   Guide for a Group Exercise[a]

Creative Thinking/Brainstorming

GOALS:

1. To identify aspects of creativity
2. To practice brainstorming

TIME REQUIRED: 1 to 1 ½ hours

MATERIALS:

1. Guidelines for effective and creative group work
2. Paper and writing instrument for each participant

PROCESS:

1. Give everyone an opportunity to read the guidelines.
2. Discuss the guidelines and clarify as needed.
3. Individually, the participants are to write down as many unusual uses as they can for one standard building brick (8.5" × 4" × 2.5"); allow 10 minutes. Emphasize that this is to be done individually. Participants should focus on only one brick and avoid listing conventional uses for bricks.
4. After their lists are made, tell them not to change or add to their lists, but they may refer to their lists during the group discussion.
5. As a group, the participants will brainstorm to produce unusual uses for the brick, using the information included in the guidelines. Allow 20 minutes. Someone should list the ideas on the board or flip chart. They may volunteer uses from their own lists. They should keep trying to produce ideas for the entire time.
6. At the end of the brainstorming, the participants will evaluate their own lists for the following aspects of creativity:

   Fluency—The total number of different uses

   Flexibility—The number of different kinds of uses

   Originality—Everyone will read the uses they have listed; as a use is named, anyone who has the same use must cross it off, including the person who read it. Continue around the group until each person's list contains uses no one else thought of; these uses are then totaled.

7. Figure the same three scores for the group list:

   Fluency—Total uses

   Flexibility—Total different kinds of uses

   Originality—Total uses not on any individual lists that were generated during brainstorming.

(continued)

TABLE 4.3 *(Continued)*

8. Ask participants to share their scores; emphasize that this is a crude measure of creativity.

9. Discuss the participants' responses to using brainstorming techniques.

---

[a] Victoria Schoolcraft developed this exercise while on the faculty of the University of Oklahoma College of Nursing.

TABLE 4.4 Interpersonal Skills Rubric (Group Process)

Instructions: Must be completed at the conclusion of group project assignment. Each student must evaluate self-behaviors that helped the group to function effectively, using the outcomes statements and rating scale provided. Each student should complete the specific questions regarding observations made while functioning within the group process.

Outcomes statements:

1. Keeps the group on task
2. Supports/praises the efforts of others
3. Encourages participation
4. Validates understanding of others/self

Rating Scale: 2 = Outstanding

1 = Demonstration of the four interpersonal skills

0 = No demonstration of the four interpersonal skills

Score: _____ (Assigned by instructor)

Complete the following questions utilizing observations/thoughts assessing the group process during the group project assignment:

1. Who emerged as group leader?
2. Was the person appointed to or assuming of the leadership role?
3. When in the process did the leader emerge?
4. Was there a power struggle within the group?
5. Who was/were the listener(s) and thinker(s) within the group?
6. Who was the one who most attempted to redirect/keep the group on task, and what did you perceive to be the motivation for the person's doing so?
7. Was there someone most apt to steer the group off topic? How and why do you think it happened?
8. Identify at least one positive and one negative interaction (regarding the process, not the topic) you learned during the group process.
9. In your assessment of the group, do you feel each member equally shared the assignment? If not, give specifics of the situation.

FINAL WORDS

After a group exercise or project is completed, the process may be evaluated using a rubric such as the one in Table 4.4. Identifying effective behaviors, as well as barriers, may aid the student's growth as an individual and as a member of a team.

FURTHER READING

Morris, D., & Turnbull, P. (2004). Issues and innovations in nursing education. *Journal of Advanced Nursing, 45*(2), 136–145.

Rauen, C. A. (2004). Simulation as a teaching strategy for nursing education and orientation in cardiac surgery. *Critical Care Nurse, 24*(3), 46–51.

Teaching Effectiveness Program Booklet. (2002). University of Oregon.

5

Planning to Give a Lecture

It has been said that a lecture is a way of getting what is in the faculty members' notes into the students' notes without the information necessarily passing through the minds of any of them. Keep this notion in mind as you prepare.

Considering how much everyone complains about lectures, it is amazing that they persist. Lydia hates giving lectures and will do anything to avoid doing one, Jim accumulates lectures as status symbols, and Marge seems convinced the students must hear each pearl of wisdom from her own lips in order to really know the material!

Many nursing faculty members give lectures because that is what the class time is called. In some academic settings, the number of lectures may contribute to fulfilling a workload commitment; or lectures may help to convey to others an idea of the expertise of faculty members. Finally, there are probably some students who will not learn material unless they hear it from the faculty. Given this range of possibilities and factors, ask the following questions before starting.

"Why am I getting ready to give a lecture?"

The most appropriate answer to any question about teaching methodology should be "because this is the most effective way to convey this material to students." If that criterion is not met by a lecture, think about some other options. Maybe a panel of nurses or patients would convey what you want the students to know. Perhaps the reading assignment is sufficient. Maybe a demonstration or observational experience is more appropriate for this topic.

"How do I feel about giving lectures?"

An instructor's nervousness will detract from a presentation. A speech course or other endeavor to learn more about public speaking may help a lecturer overcome nervousness, but maybe the reason for the discomfort relates to the first question—perhaps a lecture is not the best method to use.

"Am I able to give an effective lecture?"

Educators frequently have not considered whether they are effective at lecturing. This leads to many frightening hours for folks who really do not like to speak to groups and many boring hours for those who are required to listen. Someone may be an excellent faculty member in other aspects of the faculty appointment and yet be unable to lecture effectively. However, lecturing seems to be an activity faculty members are expected to perform. Diagnose difficulties and start to remedy them immediately.

GOALS

A lecture should offer a summary of important material unavailable to students in other forms, provide for clarification of priorities, and emphasize important content. Ideally, a lecture should not duplicate information from required readings and other resources. A lecturer should repeat things from other sources only for emphasis or explanation. A lecture should stimulate students while developing and expanding their interest and knowledge of the topic.

TOOLS

Knowledge

"Before you shoot off your mouth, be sure your brain is loaded," as a familiar saying goes. On the other hand, the entire brain does not have to be emptied into students. Perhaps the biggest shortcomings of ineffective lectures are a lack of pertinent new information and the presentation of information that is too complex for the recipients. If the faculty member lacks knowledge, this may result in a rehash of the assigned readings or a delivery of a superficial review of the content. On the other hand, if a faculty member is an expert on the content or has just finished graduate courses in the field, this sometimes leads to teaching the content in greater depth or breadth than required.

Objectives

Beforehand, decide what students should know after they have listened to the lecture. Identify what is really important for them to learn and retain. This will help in setting the objectives. Start by making a list of the concepts that need to be covered. Then decide what students need to know about these ideas. For example, do they need only to know definitions, or should they be able to apply the concepts? This will help determine the correct verbs to use in the objectives.

The objectives should be on a cognitive, psychomotor, or affective level appropriate to the course and the students. Content related to the acquisition and application of knowledge should have objectives in the cognitive realm (knowledge, comprehension, application, analysis, synthesis, and evaluation). Learning related to values, attitudes, appreciation, and personal adjustments calls for objectives in the affective realm (receiving or attending, responding, valuing, conceptualization of a value, organization of a value system, and characterization by a value or value complex). The psychomotor realm pertains to specific motor abilities.

If the course is on a lower level, the objectives should be more basic, such as definitions, identification, descriptions, lists, and so on. More advanced courses would require higher levels of objectives, such as analysis and evaluations.

Outline

Start organizing the lecture by sketching out the material to be covered in order to help the students meet the objectives. If they should be able to define a certain term, define it for them. If they are supposed to be able to analyze a certain kind of situation, tell them what is important in the situation and how they are supposed to be able to analyze it. If they need to be able to demonstrate a skill, tell them how it should be done, show them how to do it, and offer them the opportunity to practice it.

Content

After the outline is complete, begin to flesh out the content. Make sure the content flows in a logical order related to the objectives. The necessity of this aspect should seem obvious, but it is astonishing how frequently lecturers meander about, covering their content without attending to the logical order required to make sense of it.

Even though the phrase "a picture is worth a thousand words" applies literally to visual pictures, use word pictures to enhance your content. Include illustrative anecdotes from the clinical area or other aspects of life that will help to clarify and emphasize important aspects. Be sure to include these clinical and other practical examples in notes so that important points will not be forgotten.

Notes

Some faculty members have their complete lectures typed or use the printed outline view from PowerPoint or other such programs if using this technology. Typing the complete lecture word for word is not recommended because there is the danger of reading the lecture to the audience. It is better to have an outline that allows the freedom to expand or reduce the content if time becomes an issue. Using such programs as PowerPoint makes it easy to update lectures and to tailor the lecture to a specific audience. (See Tables 5.1 and 5.2.)

Practice

It is a good idea to practice the delivery of the lecture before you give it. This will make the content flow more easily as well as help time the

TABLE 5.1   Example of Detailed Lecture Notes

Testing for Creativity: Although many studies have been done to demonstrate that creativity and intelligence are not correlated, some researchers doubt the results because of their belief that what is being measured is actually intelligence rather than creativity. For example, some critics say that the "Remote Associations" test is a test of convergent thinking rather than divergent thinking. (Ask what the group thinks the difference is between intelligence and creativity.)

presentation. If you will be using equipment that is not familiar during the lecture, practice using that equipment in order to avoid frustrations.

Delivery

Voice

Make sure to articulate clearly and to speak loudly. Use a microphone if necessary. Students will miss important information if they cannot hear or are straining to listen. Refusing to use a microphone will be self-defeating.

Humor

Do not tell jokes during lectures, but use examples of situations that are humorous.

Pace

Talk at a pace that allows the students to both listen and take notes. Keep up the pace needed to cover the material without overloading the listeners. Some students may begin asking questions, indicating that they have an individual problem with the material, or the questions may pertain to material outside the purpose of the lecture. If it is obvious that many students have the same questions, answer them and try to make up lost time some other way. However, if the questions seem important to only one or two students, talk with them after class.

Closing

It helps to emphasize the most significant point of the lecture by closing with an example that illustrates important concepts. Summarize and hit the high points of the lecture.

TABLE 5.2   Example of Outlined Lecture Notes

Future research directions:

- Methods of fostering creativity
- Discriminating between intelligence and creativity
- Larger samples
- Replication (remember to give a plug for this in general as a research activity)
- Longitudinal studies

Body Language

Body language is something to consider when lecturing. Smile and let students know that the content is interesting and important. Maintain eye contact with the entire class and not just students in the first row. This takes conscious effort in the beginning but becomes easier over time. Gestures, such as touching one's hair or face, can be very distracting. Students have been known to count the number of times they observe specific behaviors rather than pay attention.

Appearance

Faculty members feel more confident about delivering a lecture when they are secure about their personal appearance. Select clothing that is comfortable, flattering, and professional. If wearing makeup, make sure it is applied in a flattering way. Check appearance before starting.

If lecturing in a large room to a large group, make certain that the background is a contrast with the color of selected clothing. If the backdrop is lightly colored, wear something colorful. If the backdrop is brown or beige, choose something lighter or darker to provide contrast. Because of the potential for the spread of germs, do not wear a uniform that was worn in the clinical area. Change clothes before coming to school.

Media

It is beyond the scope of this book to go into much detail about media software and hardware, but following are a few suggestions.

Hardware

Review the operation of the hardware prior to using it. Keep in mind that using the equipment goes with the territory of teaching. Knowing how to operate these tools is just as important as knowing how to use the equipment and skills that go along with any kind of clinical nursing.

Commercially Prepared Media

If you have rented or purchased commercially prepared media, know the media before using it. Give the students an adequate introduction before showing a film or videotape presentation so that they will know what they should be getting out of viewing the material. Afterwards, emphasize the important points and discuss how they relate to the content of the current discussion.

Handouts

Printed material should look polished and professional. If a handout has the faculty name and the name of the school on it, it should look as neat and carefully constructed as possible. When putting together a handout, keep in mind that if it contains useful information, the students may keep it for a long time.

Make sure the handout clearly conveys what is intended. Sometimes students receive handouts that contradict their readings or the lectures. If there are discrepancies that need to be cleared up with this additional data, make sure the students know which reference to use. If the handout is related to some type of process, make sure the process is clearly explained.

Producing Media

When using slides, computer programs, or overhead projections to help convey information, take time in producing media, or ask for assistance from a technician to prepare the media effectively. A "busy" slide, PowerPoint projection, or transparency is almost worse than using nothing at all. While the instructor is talking, students are struggling to decipher cryptic handwriting or to find the minute structure in the illustration.

One of the most basic rules about projected media is to keep it simple. Yet, time after time, copies are made from a standard 8 ½- by 11-inch piece of paper, and students ten or more rows away are expected to be able to distinguish line 7 from line 17.

On projected media, limit text to six or seven lines. Use large print to begin with, or find a copy machine that can increase the size of the original when it is copied. Use only single words or short phrases rather than long sentences or paragraphs.

NUTS AND BOLTS

Expert Lecturers

Attend lectures by people who the students say are good lecturers. Watch what they do and how they do it. Talk to colleagues about how they prepare and specifically how they deal with aspects of the process that are difficult.

Speech and Drama Experts

People with expertise in other fields can share tips that are useful in lecturing. For example, speech teachers and drama coaches can help formally and informally in identifying techniques that will increase effectiveness as a lecturer. These colleagues can help with voice projection or timing to convey a particular emphasis.

Coteaching

To avoid getting into competition with a colleague or ending up "suffering by comparison," work closely with that person in preparation and planning for the actual delivery of the lecture. One person may deliver some of the factual information whereas the other provides clinical illustrations or vice versa. Make a contract with each other to give and receive input about lecture style.

Evaluating Yourself

Make arrangements to have a lecture videotaped. Ask a colleague to review. This technique is helpful in evaluating verbal delivery by listening to pace, use of language, timing, and so forth.

Be certain to analyze body movements, eye contact, and other aspects of style that may contribute to or detract from effectiveness.

FINAL WORDS

Giving lectures is the most common teaching method. As with many things we all do, we tend to take it for granted and do not consider how much is involved in the process. No matter how good we are, we can probably improve our style by being aware. Remember that the student audience has paid for an education. As a role model for the profession, present knowledge with skill and style.

FURTHER READING

Bligh, D. (2000). *What is the use of lectures?* San Francisco: Jossey-Bass.

6

Planning a Successful Seminar

A seminar is a group discussion with the objective of promoting learning among the participants. A seminar enables students to learn to synthesize and use complex information. Research has demonstrated that people learn more effectively when they have an active role in the process of learning. A successful seminar is a planned discussion for the dissemination of information to provide students with practice in critical thinking.

Learning should be an active process. Introducing the seminar learning method in the classroom complements the traditional didactic lecture and makes learning more interesting. The exchange of ideas becomes an active process among students and increases student knowledge of the topic. A seminar gives the student the opportunity to take information from lectures, reading, clinical practice, and other experiences and to use that information to solve problems. We all have to learn information and skills that are not thrilling but that just have to be mastered. Whenever possible, it helps to make learning exciting. The most crucial factor directly related to the thrill of learning seems to be the desire to learn. Therefore, as faculty members, we need to look for ways to increase our students' desire to learn so that we can provide them with the information they need, and a seminar is a way to stimulate this desire while also getting the students directly involved in the teaching and learning process.

GOALS

Seminars are used to increase student involvement in the learning process. The seminar approach is useful in helping students attain high-level cognitive objectives, such as analysis, synthesis, and evaluation. This approach also promotes the achievement of affective objectives.

TOOLS

Objectives

Begin the learning experience by setting the objectives the students should accomplish. In order to write appropriate objectives, keep in mind the level of the students. A seminar is most appropriate in courses that have high-level cognitive objectives, so it is not an approach generally used in lower-division courses. Limit objectives to about four or five for a 2-hour seminar.

Objectives should provide the foundation for the outcomes of the seminar. Objectives relating only to knowledge and comprehension are usually inappropriate for seminars because such objectives require the students to only regurgitate information rather than analyze and discuss the information. Verbs such as *analyze, evaluate, explain, formulate, generalize, integrate, organize, solve,* and *synthesize* would be appropriate.

Content

The activities to be covered in the seminar should be listed in a handout. When working with students, be specific about the activities they should accomplish. Table 6.1 shows a sample seminar guide.

Some seminar activities are (1) providing a series of questions related to the objectives, (2) making a list of points drawn from the objectives for the students to discuss, or (3) including an exercise, a simulation, or other guided experience to stimulate discussion.

Process

Getting Started

The faculty member helps to start the seminar process by taking responsibility to prepare and support students. This begins with setting up ground rules for behavior. An effective way to do this is to have agreed-upon rules.

The discussion about ground rules should address the seminar start and end time and expectations for student preparation and participation and forms of presentation. It is useful to establish individual roles within a

TABLE 6.1   A Seminar Guide

Dealing with Special Group Problems

Objectives:

1. Develop an awareness of the individual and group needs that lead to special group problems.
2. Analyze the effects of selected problems.
3. Identify ways of intervening to deal with group problems.
4. Evaluate the outcomes of interventions used to deal with group problems.

Reading Assignment:

Faculty member to insert the selected assignment.

Process:

Consider the following special group problems in your discussion: monopolizing, scapegoating, silence, new members, absences, and manipulation.

1. Discuss each problem in the list using the seminar objectives.
2. How do you feel when you are in a group in which these problems exist?
3. How would you feel about being the group leader and dealing with these problems?
4. With which problems would you feel the most and the least confident in intervening?

---

group, such as timekeeper, and to divide individual work assignments. Ground rules should also look at valuing other students' opinions and maintaining confidentiality. These rules will provide structure and safety for the group discussion. See Table 6.2 for a list of possible ground rules.

If the group will meet for several seminars, it is useful to specify ground rules for the meetings. These should be printed and given to each participant.

Stimulating Discussion

Faculty can assist in stimulating discussion by leading with an open-ended question or a declarative statement. Both may help to generate discussion and highlight the contribution each person has to make. Careful planning for a seminar is essential in managing and facilitating a discussion on a specific topic. Clearly, the seminar topic and opening discussion should be relevant to the group at large.

TABLE 6.2 Seminar Ground Rules

1. The seminar will start on the hour. Everyone is expected to be present on time.

2. Each student will prepare for the seminar and will contribute to the discussion.

3. Discussion will conclude at least 15 minutes before the end of the assigned seminar time in order to permit a summary.

4. Each student will have a turn to summarize the discussion.

5. Students may not bring guests, including guest speakers, without the permission of faculty.

6. Students may not use audio or video media without the permission of faculty.

Whereas ground rules provide a foundation for student participation, advice and cueing are two strategies that may enhance student participation, reinforce behavior, and provide feedback.

Ask open-ended questions rather than questions easily answered with one- or two-word responses. For example, it would be more productive to ask, "What was the most uncomfortable experience you ever had with one of these problems?" than to ask, "Which of these problems makes you the most uncomfortable?"

When students participate and share ideas, reinforce this behavior by commenting on it. For example, "That is a good idea," "That really got us going," or "What do the rest of you think about Jan's point?"

Encouraging Appropriate Participation

Two of the most common participation problems are the students who talk too much and the students who talk too little. At the outset, set expectations about participation. Individual differences should be acknowledged. Some people are more talkative and more comfortable about talking than are others. However, both kinds of people can learn from monitoring their own and others' behavior.

Encourage those who are more comfortable talking to help by giving the quieter folks time to talk, and encourage quieter students to take advantage of this opportunity to practice in a nonthreatening situation. The principal purpose of this approach is to remind the whole group, without necessarily putting particular people on the spot, that these were the stated expectations. Emphasize that everyone in the group is responsible for the group outcome.

Limit the students from bringing outside people to the group. Outsiders change the process of a group and may interfere with the regular group members' ability to participate appropriately. Even though guest speakers who are experts on the topic may appear to be a good resource, it is usually more appropriate for the students to interview these people and share their findings than to invite them to the group. Media should be used with discretion. If used, it should be effective for stimulating discussion and should not merely consume group time.

Staying on the Topic

Another gatekeeping function is helping the group to stay on the topic. Do not get too distressed if the group goes off on a tangent. Sometimes the tangents may be more productive than what was planned. However, if the group strays from objectives and seems to be slow about getting back to the point, say something like, "OK, folks, let's get back to the objectives." Do it with a smile that conveys interest in their learning and does not give them the impression you are angry.

If the group develops a tendency to stray from the topic every time they are together, assess what they keep talking about when they ignore the seminar topics. For example, if the group also is in a clinical course together, they may continually bring up things from clinical that do not relate to the seminar goals. This may be because they do not have adequate time to deal with the impact of clinical experiences. One possible solution would be to allot some time at the beginning of each seminar to clear the air about what is on their minds. Another solution could be to find time for them to deal with such concerns outside of the seminar.

Correcting Misinformation

When students read about a particular topic for the first time, they may get an incorrect notion about what they have read. Other students may misread things or recall situations that are not accurate examples of what they are discussing. It is important to correct these erroneous ideas without seeming to put the student down for misunderstanding. If the misinformation is a common way for people to get mixed up, emphasize this so that the group can avoid the same sort of problem in the future.

Faculty might say the following: "Whoops. I think you got the variables reversed. A lot of people get independent and dependent variables mixed up. I think one reason is that in an experiment, you may be controlling the independent variable. It is hard to think of something that is being controlled as being independent. However, outside the experiment, that variable is not being controlled, and we think it affects the dependent variable in some way."

A straightforward explanation conveys important information and keeps the students' energy focused on meeting the objectives rather than on trying to regurgitate definitions. In a situation such as the one just described, follow up with some examples and help the group to identify which variable is which, in order to increase their confidence in dealing with the material.

Sometimes, a student has a vested interest in the piece of misinformation. The student may become caught up in trying to defend the information for personal reasons.

Although it is likely that most instructors have distressed students inappropriately, it sometimes may actually promote learning to encourage students to be distressed about not knowing the correct answer. For example, if there is a lot of controversy about the right answer, refrain from providing the answer and ask the students to look further for the correct answers and bring them back to the seminar.

Drawing to Closure

Closure is another ground rule to establish. It helps to have a summary touching on the high points in the discussion or significant realizations the group has reached. For the first seminar, give the students an idea of what should be included in the summary. After that, continue to take this responsibility for a few meetings, and then ask a student to do it. The summary helps to solidify the understandings gained from the discussion. It can also provide a direction for further discussions of the same topic or subsequent topics.

NUTS AND BOLTS

Leadership

Faculty members take on leadership responsibilities in a seminar with inexperienced students. Leadership in a seminar takes the form of facilitating the students through the process described earlier in this chapter. With advanced students, expect them to take some of the leadership responsibilities. However, the faculty member has the ultimate responsibility for helping to make this a positive learning experience.

If the students will be responsible for facilitating seminar discussions, give them some guidance to get started. For example, assign a reading about the seminar process, or review the process as it is described in this chapter.

When students have leadership responsibilities, decide who will be responsible for each seminar. Generally, two students work together. They can share the work for preparation as well as the tasks of facilitating the group. More than two students is inappropriate because it is unrealistic to expect a group to function with the leadership responsibilities spread so thin.

Faculty members occasionally have unrealistic expectations of the sophistication of students in leadership roles. They may expect students to confront and deal with complex problems of participation without any faculty assistance. When there are problems either within one meeting or within the group as a whole, the faculty member needs to step in and help to bring the problems into the open for discussion.

Evaluation

In some situations, it may be appropriate to evaluate and grade seminars. Evaluation may include assessment of the students' meeting the objectives adequately in relation to content as well as evaluation of the process itself. The evaluation may be as basic as acknowledging that each objective was met and how. Develop an evaluation tool that integrates the content and the process. An example is given in Table 6.3.

For courses in which seminars constitute a major portion of the course activity, attach a grade to the evaluation. Generally, this is done when the course has important objectives that are met only through the seminar. A seminar grade is also more common when there is a significant weight placed on group process as a part of the framework of the curriculum.

If evaluating and grading the seminars in the course, be sure to keep the course objectives and their relative weights in mind. For example, if the seminars deal with major content, and group process is very significant, both content and process should be given significant weight in determining

TABLE 6.3   Seminar Evaluation Guide

Content:

1. Seminar objectives were met.

   - 100% of objectives were met.
   - 90% of objectives were met.
   - 70% of objectives were met.
   - Less than 70% of objectives were met.

2. Correct information was shared.

   - 100% of information was complete and accurate.
   - 90% of information was complete and accurate.
   - 70% of information was complete and accurate.
   - Less than 70% of information was complete and accurate.

3. Appropriate references were used.

   - Assigned reading plus other resources
   - Assigned reading plus one other resource
   - Assigned reading only

4. Useful examples and experiences were shared.

   - Many examples and anecdotes
   - Some examples and anecdotes
   - Few examples and anecdotes
   - No examples or anecdotes

Process:

1. The seminar started on time.
2. All members participated.
3. Participation was appropriate (i.e., no silent members, no monopolizing).
4. The group stayed on the assigned topic.
5. If problems were present, the group dealt with them.
6. A summary was presented.
7. The seminar ended on time.

the students' course grades. In other situations, less may be expected of the students and less weight given to any evaluation and grade.

With students who are less experienced in seminar activities, the faculty member may start by doing the total evaluation. As the students gain more experience, they can begin to participate in the evaluation and eventually in the grading.

Expect more from the outset from students who are experienced in seminars and grade them accordingly. With inexperienced seminar participants or with a new group, grade more leniently in the first few meetings. Try to be realistic about what your students can handle, given their backgrounds.

When students participate in the grading, allot different percentages to how much the faculty member and the students contribute to the final grade. Separate the process grade from the content grade. For example, in one situation, the students and faculty each contributed one-third of the grade based on the achievement of content. The last third was contributed only by faculty and was based on the faculty evaluation of the group's ability to evaluate their own process. The formula is in Table 6.4.

If formula outlined in Table 6.4 is used, main control over the grade is left with the faculty, although the students can certainly influence the grade. Part of the students' evaluation could include some points on their own evaluation of their group process. This approach is especially appropriate in courses where group process and change are important aspects. Because the faculty member evaluates the students on their ability to recognize and try to correct their problems, students can partially improve their grade if they are honest and insightful in their self-evaluation.

Trying to grade individuals in a seminar is very complex. Although, on the face of it, it seems a good idea to evaluate each individual separately, it is very difficult to do so fairly. In order to give some credit for individual preparation for seminar, require a bibliography card on the assigned reading, or give a short quiz over the reading assignment. Remember that the written word requires more time to read, comment on, and grade. Another strategy that may be more appealing is setting aside time in the seminar for the students to share their bibliography cards or having the students grade each other's quizzes and use the information when they proceed with their discussion.

TABLE 6.4   Group-Grade Calculation Formula

Content: a = faculty grade; b = student grade

Evaluation process: c = faculty grade

Seminar grade = (a + b + c) divided by 3

Example: (93 + 95 + 98) divided by 3 = 95.33

FINAL WORDS

Seminars can be effective ways to facilitate achievement of high-level objectives. Careful planning and facilitation lead to a successful seminar. Seminar participation assists in developing critical thinking skills and understanding the dynamics of group process. This method of teaching allows for an active and shared responsibility toward creating a goal-oriented learning experience.

FURTHER READING

Stiles, A. S., Johnson, R. K., Trigg, B. K., & Fowler, G. (2004). Cooperative learning: The ugly, the bad, and the good. *Nurse Educator, 29,* 97–98.

Xakellis, G. C., Richner, S., & Stevenson, F. (2005). Comparison of knowledge acquired by students in small group seminars with and without a formal didactic component. *Medical Student Education, 37,* 27–29.

7

Course Design, Implementation, and Evaluation

The more time and effort invested into designing a course, the fewer problems when the course is implemented. Even a fairly standard course, such as a medical-surgical nursing course, will need work toward putting it together in a logical and useful way.

The first time a faculty member is asked to teach, that faculty member usually is not expected to design the course. However, the new faculty member will soon need to know how to do this. Rather than copying what another faculty member designed for another curriculum, know the principles involved.

It is easier to describe this process in the order that will eventually show up in a course syllabus. Start by listing the content that should go into the course and write the course description later. Course descriptions and course objectives need to be approved by the curriculum committee, so do not make changes unless you have approval.

GOALS

Effective course design facilitates presentation of content. Attention to design makes it possible to acquaint students from the outset with the direction and expectations of the course.

TOOLS

Curriculum Context

Theoretical Model
Whether or not the curriculum is based on a well-known model, there is a framework around which it is organized. Most schools have a content

map. The elements of the model, content map, and framework dictate the organization of each of the courses. Before trying to design the course, understand the context.

In many nursing curricula, the major organizing concepts are person (or humanity), environment, health (or health and illness), and nursing. To some extent, each course in the curriculum reflects these concepts, advances the students' understanding of them individually, and promotes the students' grasp of the interrelationships.

Usually, the organizing concepts are defined in the school's philosophy. Although there are diverse definitions, there are also similarities in which aspects of these concepts are described. *Person* is described as an individual, perhaps in terms of interactions with others. The person may be described as an independent, dependent, or interdependent organism. If the school is part of a sectarian college, the relationship of the person to a higher power may be included.

Environment describes the milieu in which the person and nursing intersect. *Health* or *health and illness* will be described in terms of the impact of nursing intervention. *Nursing* is described in relation to the scope of practice and its place as a profession.

Placement

The year in which the students are expected to take the course determines the complexity of the course design. Courses early in the curriculum will be based on simpler objectives. Generally, courses should move from the simple to the complex and from the normal to the abnormal.

Prerequisites

The course must be placed so that students will have completed appropriate prerequisites in order to be able to understand the new content. If the requirement is for the students to know complex pharmacology, but complex pharmacology is not to be taught in the course, schedule the course after students have taken the appropriate courses. By the same token, do not repeat content or assignments already tackled in a prerequisite course unless there is a new application that students need to learn.

If the course is meant to be prerequisite to other courses, make sure to include the content students will need when they get to the other courses.

For example, if the course is supposed to prepare students to develop teaching care plans and they will not get this information elsewhere, make room for that content and the application of teaching and learning principles.

Strands

Another common feature of nursing curricula is strands or threads that are woven throughout and help to support the major concepts. These strands often include the following: nutrition; pharmacology; professionalism; individual, family, and group; acute, rehabilitative, and chronic care; hospital and community settings; and primary, secondary, and tertiary prevention. These strands vary according to the other organizing elements in the framework, but whatever they are within the curriculum, consider how to incorporate them into the course. Not every course will include all of the strands. For example, nutrition and pharmacology might not be found in a course on nursing trends and issues. However, the strand of professionalism would be the predominant theme in that course.

Format

Usually, there will be an established format to follow. Look at the way other courses are set up, especially how the syllabi for similar courses are organized. This will establish the pattern for designing the course.

An abbreviated sample of a syllabus format is shown in Table 7.1. In addition to the introductory information furnished in the sample, attach guides for the course's required assignments and evaluation tools.

Having consistent patterns helps in preparing self-study reports for state approval as well as for reports by the Commission on Collegiate Nursing Education (CCNE) or National League for Nursing Accrediting Commission (NLNAC).

Course Description

The course description should give a concise overview of the course, describe the principal focus, and identify the major teaching methodologies. An example would be the following:

Nursing Concepts 1. Introduction to the systematic use of the nursing process in selected clinical settings. Focus is on the individual with major

TABLE 7.1   Format for a Course Syllabus

Beta University Alpha School of Nursing

N321 Psychiatric Mental Health Nursing

Course Description: Focus is on the use of the nursing process with acutely ill psychiatric patients in an inpatient setting. Emphasis is on the use of self in promoting therapeutic nurse–patient relationships. Experience is limited to working with adults.

Placement in Curriculum: Junior standing; prerequisites are N232 and N237.

Conceptual Framework: Psychiatric or mental health nurses use interpersonal communication skills and the nursing process to assist persons who are temporarily dependent due to severe psychiatric or emotional problems interfering with their mental health. Strands addressed in this course include research, pharmacology, professionalism, individual/family/group, acute/rehabilitative/chronic care, hospital/community settings, and primary/secondary/tertiary prevention.

Course Objectives: At the end of this course, the student will be able to

1. Describe the use of the nursing process with psychiatric patients
2. Identify and implement therapeutic nursing interventions for use with adult psychiatric patients
3. Differentiate between nursing practice with psychiatric patients and the practice of other mental health workers

Required Text: Keltner, N., & Schweche, L. (2003). *Psychiatric Nursing* (4th ed.). St. Louis, Mosby.

Evaluation and Grading: The theory grade will be determined by the student's performance on two tests and a comprehensive final examination. The student's clinical performance and the written nursing care study will determine the clinical grade. Students will be formally evaluated at midterm and at the end of the term using the evaluation tool included in the syllabus.

Theory:	Test 1, 15%
	Test 2, 15%
	Final, 20%
Clinical:	Performance, 35%
	Case study, 15%

Students must receive a passing grade in both clinical and in theory before the grades are averaged for the course grade. A failure in either part of the course constitutes a failure in the course.

(continued)

TABLE 7.1   *(Continued)*

Content:	Assigned Reading:
Conceptual Framework	Chapters 1–3
Therapeutic Use of Self	Chapters 4, 10, 13
Nursing Process	Chapters 11–12
Patterns of Anxiety	Chapters 29–31
Depression and Elation	Chapters 34–36

emphasis on alterations in fluid/electrolyte balance, acid/base status, and blood composition. Needs in the following areas are addressed: comfort and sleep, oxygenation, nutrition, elimination, mobility, grieving, aging, and dying. Practical laboratory experience includes acquisition of health-assessment techniques and clinical experience in hospital and extended care facilities.

This course description would be appropriate for course materials, but some colleges and universities require shorter descriptions for the catalog. If shortening the description is necessary, try to make it convey as much as possible in the words allowed. The original is 69 words long. It would be possible to write a shorter version, with only 42 words, without losing anything significant:

Nursing Concepts 1. Introduction to the systematic use of the nursing process with individuals experiencing alterations in fluid/electrolytes and acid/base levels, blood composition, and human-functioning needs. Practical experience includes acquisition of health-assessment techniques and clinical experience in hospital and extended care facilities.

Neither of these descriptions constitutes timeless prose, but both do a fair job of telling a prospective student or anyone else something about the course. Even a novice or outsider could probably grasp the meaning of the words used in this context.

Course Objectives

The objectives should proceed logically from the course description and should be written with consideration for the elements listed earlier under the section on curriculum context. Because the course description in the example is obviously for a beginning-level course, write objectives on the lower cognitive levels pertaining more to knowledge, comprehension, and application. Some examples are available in Table 7.2. The objectives in the table are written in measurable behavioral terms. More specific objectives can be drawn from these for each class or clinical experience.

Content

Organize the content in the order reflected by the objectives or in the chronological order in which it will be covered. Make sure the content is on the appropriate level. As in the example, if blood disorders need to be addressed, limit the depth of information for a beginning-level course.

Reading Assignments

The following chapter deals with selecting texts and making reading assignments, but these tasks also need to be considered in planning the course.

TABLE 7.2   Course Objectives

At the conclusion of this course, the student will be able to:

1. Describe each step in the nursing process
2. Demonstrate beginning ability to use the nursing process in working with individual clients
3. Apply the nursing process in working with individuals with alterations in fluid/electrolyte balance, acid/base status, and blood composition
4. Use the nursing process in addressing needs in the areas of human functioning: comfort/sleep, oxygenation, nutrition, elimination, and mobility
5. Identify and respond to nursing care needs for individuals who are grieving, aging, and dying
6. Demonstrate competent and safe use of health assessment techniques

If a textbook has been chosen, consider putting the course content in the same order as in the book. This will make the book easier for the students to use.

Evaluation and Grading of Students

Decide how to evaluate the students' achievement of the course objectives. Relate these methods to the level of the course objectives. The course should include a reasonable amount of work for the credits assigned to the course. A combination of major and minor assignments and examinations is advised. The details of selecting and using these tools are described in later chapters, but include the relevant information for the students in the course syllabus.

Teaching Methodology

Determine the most effective means to help the students learn the content and use the processes included in the course. If objectives are mostly in the cognitive realm and on the levels of knowledge, comprehension, and application, the lecture method is most efficient. If dealing with higher cognitive levels of analysis, synthesis, and evaluation or if dealing with objectives in the affective domain, methods such as seminar will better enable the students to practice meeting such objectives. Psychomotor objectives can best be met by the students' having practiced laboratory or clinical experiences. Clinical experiences in most nursing courses will provide an opportunity for addressing objectives at different levels in any domain, but the expectations will be simpler in the first courses as contrasted with the more advanced courses in the curriculum.

Course Evaluation

Course evaluation is the responsibility of the faculty with input from the students. Plan for the evaluation of the course from the start and fit it into the system used by the school. If there are components of the course that need special evaluation, add them to the tool being used within the program. Be sure to allow class time for students to evaluate the course and the faculty who teach it.

In addition to the students' evaluations, keep a log or file of faculty perceptions of the components of the course. For example, after giving a lecture, an instructor may decide that the content was too complex. Write that down with ideas of how to change in the future. Use this evaluation of the course and the summary of the students' evaluations to determine what needs to be changed and how.

NUTS AND BOLTS

Guest Speakers or Experts

As a new faculty member, you may be responsible for the majority of the work entailed in implementing the course. However, do not hesitate to enlist the help of other nursing faculty members for some classes as well as practicing nurses outside the faculty. For example, invite a nursing faculty member who specializes in ethics to lecture on ethical implications within the scope of the course.

There is a lot of work involved in developing lectures for 15 weeks of class. Although instructors teach from the area of expertise, it still takes time to put together cohesive lectures that will help the students meet the objectives. Bring in a local expert for a lecture if need be. For example, if you are teaching a course in psychiatric nursing and have little experience in the treatment of substance abuse, invite a clinical nursing specialist in the field to lecture on this topic.

Before asking a guest to lecture on a topic, ascertain that person's ability to speak in public. A lot of people are nervous about speaking to a group. Their anxiety may result in failing to address objectives. They might run over the allotted time or run too short, leaving the students in a bind either way. If possible, listen to the potential guest speaker ahead of time. If this cannot be arranged, find someone trusted to evaluate the prospective speaker.

Sometimes, it will not be possible to validate speaking ability ahead of time, so be prepared for some of the more predictable problems. The first way to avoid trouble is to contact the guest well in advance. Discuss what that person is to address and share the lecture objectives in writing. Suggest another brief chat prior to the lecture so that the person can tell you what is planned. Give the guest, in writing, the ground rules, such as the starting time for the class, when to give breaks (if appropriate), and when to end the class. Discuss how the guest will handle student questions, including when to get back to covering the planned material. Also find out in advance if the guest will require any media support.

Once you and the guest have agreed to the parameters, send a letter that validates the plans. Include all the particulars, including equipment that will be available. Give explicit directions about the location and parking.

A week or so before the guest will be present, send an email or make a telephone call to touch base and find out if there are any questions or problems. Validate that the guest will be able to find the classroom or know where to meet you so that you can go to the classroom together. If possible, it is courteous to meet the guest a little before the class time. Go to your office and share some refreshments or otherwise make the guest feel welcome and at home. Usually faculty will not be in a position to offer the guest any monetary remuneration for this service, so little personal gestures and attention to details can do a lot to show genuine gratitude for the expert speaker's contribution.

When introducing the guest to the students, share the guest's credentials and explain why he or she was chosen to lecture. Then turn the class over. Usually, things will go fine, even if the guest strays a bit or does not address every objective. Sometimes, if the class is large, discipline problems may occur. Remind students to be respectful and professional.

After the class, attend to details that show gratitude. Within a day or two, follow up with a note or letter thanking the guest for helping. If possible, address something specific about the presentation to make the thank-you personal. For example, you may write, "Your description of the teenage patient withdrawing from alcohol was especially powerful and instructive." After the lecture, evaluate the guest to decide whether to make the same invitation in the future.

Organizing

No matter how helpful this or any other book may be in helping to prepare and present a course, seasoned colleagues on the faculty will be useful resources. Administrative or clerical staff members are also invaluable in helping to figure out how things really work. The responsibilities of a course coordinator may vary from school to school. The following responsibilities may be those of either faculty or other people. Figure out how the following tasks are accomplished.

Requesting classrooms
Arranging for clinical sites
Having your syllabus typed and duplicated
Selecting texts
Putting readings on reserve in the library
Securing audiovisual software and hardware
Arranging for guest speakers
Preparing your own lectures
Constructing tests and having them printed
Arranging for machine grading of tests
Grading assignments
Arranging for course and faculty evaluation
Distributing midterm grade deficiencies
Counseling students with problems in the course
Reporting final grades
Developing proficiency examinations

Institutional Policies

Be informed about institutional policies about the presentation of courses. These can usually be found in the catalog or a policy manual. Some of the issues affected by such policies are listed below. Check on these to see if there is an official policy before making a decision.

Beginning and ending dates of the course
Class times (starting, stopping, and breaks)
Official holidays
Canceling or rescheduling classes
Numerical values of letter grades
Auditors in class
Dates for dropping or withdrawing from courses
Recipients of deficiency notices
Restrictions on and removal of incomplete grade
Recipient of official grade reports

Examination policies covering the following:

Required exams
Makeup exams
Time of final exam

Credit by proficiency examination
Grievances

FINAL WORDS

Although designing a course may not be required of a faculty member immediately, do learn by watching how it has been done. Eventually this responsibility will be part of a new faculty member's role. Although it is challenging at first, most faculty enjoy having this chance to be creative and to share their knowledge and expertise.

FURTHER READING

Billings, C. M., & Halstead, J. A. (2005). *Teaching in nursing: A guide for faculty* (2nd ed.). Philadelphia: Saunders.

8

Textbook and Reading-Assignment Selection

The information available in print is expanding at ever-increasing rates. In the twenty-first century, the knowledge base in all sciences and professions is expanding exponentially!

The Cumulative Index to Nursing and Allied Health reviews and indexes approximately 1500 journals. With new journals cropping up each year, it is difficult for nursing professionals to keep up with the literature in their own fields of nursing, let alone in all areas of nursing practice.

Depending on the editorial policies of a given book publisher or journal, what is in print may have been written 1 to 3 years earlier. Because the lag time from writing to publishing is usually greater for books than for journals, what appears in journals may be more current or accurate. Actually, even though there are some areas more prone to rapid change than others, textbooks are probably more complete and comprehensive than ever before. Many new editions of books include computer disks, test banks, laboratory manuals, and other helpful supplements.

In any text, the author or editor must make choices about what can be included and in what depth the topics will be handled. An author also decides about the model or organizational framework used to present the content. These decisions must be considered when choosing textbooks for students.

GOALS

The principal goal for reading material is to provide the students with accurate information on a given topic. In addition, faculty members must identify a reasonable number of reading assignments so that students will be able to complete them.

TOOLS

Evaluating Prospective Texts

Process Criteria

Before reviewing any texts, set the criteria to evaluate your options. In addition to coverage of the general content, set standards for expectations in specific areas. Other concerns will be with the way the material is presented, such as whether it follows a particular theorist's model, or whether it is aimed at the level required for the class.

Table 8.1 includes a format that can be used to evaluate a text. The form may be used to evaluate a book in any clinical area of nursing. Rating the elements with a Likert scale from 0 for "Unsatisfactory" to 5 for "Excellent" may be useful when comparing similar textbooks. Other items may be evaluated with dichotomous options of "Yes" or "No."

Content Criteria

In addition to the general evaluation, prepare a list of topics in your area that will be assessed. As an example, Table 8.2 shows a content checklist for evaluating psychiatric nursing texts.

If more than one faculty member is evaluating the books for possible adoption, prepare the evaluation criteria together. Decide ahead of time how differences of opinion will be resolved about which book to adopt. Following the evaluation of the textbooks, share your evaluations and decide on the textbooks that will be adopted.

Date of Publication

Although date of publication is a factor to consider, some books that are a few years older are still better than the ones that have just been published.

Cost

Faculty members often have no idea of the cost of the texts that they are reviewing for their courses. This is a significant factor to consider when your students are already spending so much on books. If you are choosing between two or more texts, and they are about equal, choose the least expensive book. If the book is available in a cheaper paperback version, ensure that the bookstore orders that format.

TABLE 8.1   Textbook Evaluation Form

Name of textbook _____

Publisher _____

Cost _____

Author_____

Publication date_____

Replaces text_____

General:

_____Conceptual framework harmonious with ours

_____Comprehensive

_____Emphasis on nursing models

_____Approach to nursing process consistent with ours

_____Definitions consistent with our terminology

_____Builds on prerequisite content

_____Aimed at students in upper division

_____Internally consistent

_____Nonsexist language

_____Useful index

Format:

_____Objectives given

_____Clear chapter introductions

_____Theory is current; recent reference citations

_____Nursing research is discussed and used

_____Clear examples are given to illustrate important points

_____Significant issues are emphasized

_____Headings enhance ease of finding material

_____Important content is highlighted

_____Photographs, tables, graphs, and diagrams

_____Summaries are succinct and recap important points

Readability:

_____Size and style of print promote ease of reading

_____Narrative style enhances reading

(continued)

TABLE 8.1 *(Continued)*

_____Appropriate reading level for course

_____Readability score

Instructional aids:

Instructor's manual available

Student workbook available

Media available

   Specify types_____

Test-item bank available

_____Book form _____Computer software

Comments:

TABLE 8.2 Content Checklist

Psychiatric/Mental Health Nursing Text

Diagnosis-Related Content:

_____Affective disorders

   _____Bipolar disorder

   _____Major depression

_____Anxiety disorders

   _____Acute

   _____Chronic

_____Death and dying

_____Dissociative disorders

_____Grief

_____Organic mental disorders

_____Paranoid disorder

_____Personality disorders

   _____Antisocial personality

   _____Borderline personality

_____Psychosis

   _____Acute

   _____Schizophrenia

(continued)

TABLE 8.2 *(Continued)*

_____Self-destructive behavior

_____Sexual dysfunction

_____Substance abuse

_____Violent behavior

    _____Victims of violence

    _____Violent clients

Contributory Content:

_____Community mental health

_____Crisis intervention

_____Family components

_____Historical perspectives

_____Legal and ethical issues

_____Life span considerations

_____Psychoactive drugs

_____Psychosocial development

_____Research

_____Social and cultural aspects

_____Therapeutic approaches

    _____Alternative therapies

    _____Traditional therapies

_____Therapeutic groups

_____Therapeutic interpersonal communication

Other content included:

Different Versions

Some authors have more than one version of their work. For example, Polit and Beck together are the authors of both *Essentials of Nursing Research* and *Nursing Research*. The first book is intended for consumers of nursing research, such as undergraduates, and the second book, written with Hungler, is for producers of research, such as graduate students.

Although not published by the same authors, there are books within each specialty area of nursing that are intended for one level of student or another. Hockenberry, Wilson, Winkelstein, and Kline have published *Wong's Nursing Care of Infants and Children,* and Whaley and Wong have published *Essentials of Pediatric Nursing.* The former is comprehensive and is intended for baccalaureate programs. The latter is more appropriate for associate degree programs. Make sure to select the right book in the first place when you begin the evaluation process.

Amount of Use

When selecting a book, ascertaining the proportion of the book you will actually be able to use is important. If you can assign at least 60% to 75%, it is probably reasonable to consider the book. However, if there are many chapters that will not be assigned by you and that probably will not be assigned by other faculty in the program either, it may be unreasonable to require students to purchase the text.

If the program has more than one course with similar content, the same type of text may be required. For example, students may have one course dealing with fundamental medical-surgical nursing early in the program and then another course later dealing with complex medical-surgical content. If the two courses require the same kind of text, the faculty involved in the courses should collaborate on selecting texts. It may be necessary to have two different books, such as a text on fundamentals and a more comprehensive medical-surgical text. However, if the students are going to use the comprehensive type of text in both courses, the faculty should agree on one text rather than require the students to invest in two books with the same content.

Supplementing With Journal Readings

As long as typical undergraduate students are making an investment in their textbooks, these books should be used as much as possible to satisfy the reading requirements for the class. However, there are some topics that texts may neglect to cover in a suitable fashion. When this happens, readings from other sources are quite appropriate.

Also, there are some courses for which no text is readily available. If you are going to use journal articles, make sure you use them with discretion. The details of weighing text and journal assignments are covered in the next section.

NUTS AND BOLTS

Procedures for Text Review

Identifying Potential Texts

There are a number of ways to find out about new texts, such as through publishers' ads in journals and other media, book reviews in journals, contacts with publishers' representatives on campus, or meetings and contacts with colleagues. Write to the publishers of nursing texts and ask to be put on their mailing and e-mail lists for catalogs and other book announcements. Publishers may also provide e-mail alerts to their mailing lists regarding topics of interest. Browsing the publisher's Internet Web sites is another easy way to identify potential texts.

Securing Books for Review

Some publishers will automatically send a new edition of a book that has been adopted for a class. Sales representatives will call or visit the school to get lists of the faculty members and their specialties in order to send them books.

Faculty members who want a specific book can get review copies of texts by calling or writing to the publisher of the book. Use their response cards for this or print your correspondence on the school's letterhead. Publishers usually want to know the name of the course, how many times a year the course is offered, and the average enrollment of students. They also may want to know what book you currently use, who will participate in the selection, and when a decision will be made.

Usually, it is possible to get a complimentary copy of a text that can be kept whether or not the book is adopted. If it is a specialty book not usually used as a text, faculty may only be able to review it for a set time if it is not adopted. If the text is adopted, faculty will probably be able to keep it without charge.

Review Timetable

Set a specific time period during which textbooks will be reviewed for adoption, or review them on an ongoing basis. A lot of texts are published in the early part of the year, so as to be hot off the press when faculty are making their decisions for the coming academic year. Be sure that there is enough time for the bookstore to get the copies for the students. Sometimes a book is so well received that distributors run out of copies, and the bookstore may not be able to get copies until after the term starts.

Rules of Thumb in Assigning Readings

Read the Assigned Readings

Taking the time to read the assigned texts carefully is a very simple but vital task. If a chapter in a text or an article has a certain title, sometimes it is taken for granted that the topic is covered adequately. However, the piece may have one of the following shortcomings:

- It neglects important points.
- It does not emphasize priorities.
- It includes too much detail.
- It repeats or contradicts other readings.

Amount of Reading

A rule of thumb for assignments to be completed outside of class is to allow for 2 to 3 hours of reading per week per credit hour. For example, 2 hours $\times$ 3 credits = 6 hours per week of outside work.

Accessibility

Obviously, assignments from the students' textbooks will be the most accessible. When readings are assigned outside the students' texts, consider how available these will be. Although it is legitimate to want to encourage students to use the library, there may be better ways to accomplish that goal than to require them to go to the library when their texts will suffice.

Evaluate the holdings and the policies of the library the students will use. If you will be providing your own copy of a book or article, find out how the library handles these materials. If you provide photocopied material, make sure that copyright laws are followed.

Copyright Compliance

Reproduction of copyrighted material without prior permission of the copyright owner is an issue for the academic community. Remember that as in other applications of the law, "Ignorance is no defense." As an educator, you are expected to understand the copyright law and indulge only in "fair use" of copied material.

To begin with, indiscriminate copying of published works deprives authors of control of their written work as well as income. Although the law is somewhat generous to teachers as to what constitutes fair use, it is important that all aspects of the law be followed. It is essential that all faculty members have a copy of *Questions and Answers on Copyright for the Campus Community,* which is published by the National Association of College Stores, Inc., the Association of American Publishers, Inc., and the Association of American University Presses, Inc.

Some publishers of journals sell reprints of articles expected to be of continuing use. They are not likely to give permission to make copies. In this situation, request that the library or the administration purchase reprints, or establish this as a required purchase the students will make when they buy their textbooks.

Unique Contribution

When choosing assignments, make sure not to assign repetitious material. Faculty members sometimes assign a three- or four-page article when only a small portion conveys something different from or more than other reading available in the text.

Contradictions

Another reason to read the assignments before the students is to validate that they are in harmony with one another. If there are real or apparent contradictions between readings, clarify for students which account is the one they need to learn, or help them to understand that there are differences of opinion on the issue.

FINAL WORDS

Selecting appropriate textbooks and reading assignments is a key activity in teaching effectively. This is one of the indirect ways in which faculty influence students' learning. Use discretion in the choices and maximize the results of the students' reading time.

FURTHER READING

Questions and answers on copyright for the campus community. (2003). Available from the National Association of College Stores, Inc., 500 East Lorain Street, Oberlin, OH 44074-1294.

9

Designing and Grading a Major Assignment

What do students get from doing assignments? Ideally an assignment will enhance learning. Some students seem frustrated and overwhelmed by any assignment, but hopefully the assignments will be challenging for those who can handle them yet manageable for those who may not be fully up to the challenge.

An assignment should fit within the context of the course, especially in terms of the course objectives. For example, an assignment would not be appropriate in a lower-division course, with primarily lower cognitive levels of objectives, which can be met by listening to lectures, viewing media, and reading. Because it is typical for upper-division and graduate courses to have higher-level objectives, students in those courses need experiences exceeding those in lower-division courses. It is helpful in evaluating students to give them assignments that permit them to demonstrate higher-order cognitive skills.

GOALS

A major assignment should be used to allow the student to demonstrate accomplishment of high-level objectives. Such an assignment permits the evaluation of learning, which is not easily evaluated objectively.

DEFINITION OF A MAJOR ASSIGNMENT

The qualities that differentiate between major and minor assignments are (1) depth and breadth of content involved, (2) time required for completion, and (3) the amount of credit attached to the evaluation of the finished product. When any of these qualities is substantial, the assignment is defined as major.

One determination of how much substantive work is involved in fulfilling an assignment is the amount of work required outside of class. A general rule for determining a reasonable amount of work outside of class is a ratio of 2 or 3 hours to each hour spent in class. A formula for calculating amount of work outside of class would be: number of credit hours $\times$ 2 (or 3) hours $\times$ number of weeks in quarter or semester.

Thus, for a three-credit semester course, the students could be expected to complete 90 to 135 hours of work outside of class over the course of the semester: 3×2 (or 3) $\times 15 = 90$ (or 135) hours outside of class. This outside work would include all the required reading and the preparation of assignments necessary for the students to meet the requirements of the course. If a great deal of reading were required, the time remaining to devote to an assignment would be limited. By the same token, a major assignment would limit the time for outside reading.

A major assignment is usually designed to give students an opportunity to choose one area to study to a greater extent, in terms of increased depth or breadth, or both. For example, in a graduate course on nursing theory, students may be assigned to study one theory in depth. In an undergraduate course, students may be given an assignment to identify ten different interventions to reach the same outcome.

The amount of work involved should be directly related to the weight the grade on the assignment will carry in determining the course grade. For example, an assignment that will take one-third of the allotted time outside of class to complete could be rewarded with a major portion of the course grade.

TYPES OF ASSIGNMENTS

Major Paper

Purposes

A major paper, usually 10 to 12 pages, not only allows students to demonstrate abilities with higher cognitive objectives, but also permits them the opportunity to practice putting their ideas in writing. A paper is particularly useful when your aims relate to critical thinking, analysis, or organizational skills.

Preparation

The time that is required for students to prepare a paper may be extensive, depending on your expectations. There are two different approaches to determining the content requirements of the paper. A student-centered paper includes a description or analysis of something the student did, as with nursing-care plans. The other major type is a concept-centered paper in which the student investigates a concept or issue in depth, such as a paper on a professional issue or a physiological or psychosocial principle. A paper based on the student's own activities usually requires less time in gathering information, but more time in organizing and analyzing. A paper dealing with a concept or issue requires more investigation of the literature and also calls for organization and analysis.

The complexity of a paper is related to the extent of the literature search required to support the student's ideas. It takes time for the student to locate appropriate resources and read the selections. For students less experienced with the process of writing a paper, each reference may take up to 3 hours to locate, read, and incorporate into the paper. Students who have had experience have often learned ways of simplifying some of these steps, but it is a good idea to assess their abilities in this regard. This process is dealt with at greater length in chapter 14.

Although the situation varies, depending on the complexity of the ideas involved, an average student may take an hour or more to compose one page of text. If the student is conscientious in writing, he or she will probably complete at least one or two drafts before the final copy. This means it could take a student between 10 and 20 hours to compose a 10-page paper, apart from the literature search and reading time.

Grading

Develop a list of evaluation criteria such as those in Table 9.1 and use the list as a grading guide. Objectivity in grading is important, but even so, there will always be a certain degree of subjectivity.

Major papers take a long time to grade, and nursing students often concentrate on getting the assignment done, so they do not spend much time trying to make what they write interesting. Because of this, carefully consider whether a major paper is appropriate for the course requirements. If this will be a valuable way to assess students' achievement of objectives, be sure to have the papers submitted early enough to allow plenty of time for grading.

TABLE 9.1 Evaluation Criteria for a Major Paper

Evaluation Criteria	
Assessment	
Data is logically summarized	5
Significant data are identified	5
Planning	
State appropriate outcomes	15
Identify three top priorities	10
State criteria for evaluation of outcomes	10
Implementation	
Identify interventions to accomplish the three top priorities for care	20
Cite references for interventions	10
Describe one unique intervention	5
Evaluation	
Evaluate outcomes for three top priorities	5
Evaluate own performance of care	. 5
Style and Format	
Paper is typewritten, double-spaced	3
APA format is used for references	3
Correct grammar and spelling are used	4
Total points	100

Experienced faculty members know that the worst papers take the most time to grade. The sentence structure, grammar, and organization may be difficult to follow. Some students have difficulty with what content they should include, no matter how clearly it was described in the requirements.

Students who do poorly on the paper will probably feel that they have spent a lot of time on it and may think that they should get a better grade simply because of the amount of time involved. Never doubt the time students claim they spend, but point out that the product is what they are being graded on.

Occasionally, a student will submit a paper that is exceptional in that it is thoughtfully done and well written. However, that does not happen as often as one would like.

Projects

Purposes

A project offers the opportunity for application of knowledge in a practical situation. Some examples familiar to nursing educators are community studies, teaching projects, health screening, research critiques, and research proposals. Although such assignments may be done outside of class time, in some cases they may be done during clinical time for a course.

Preparation

Although a project may be completed within the allotted course time, the requirements may necessitate students' completing some work outside of scheduled time. Time must be spent orienting and supervising students involved in projects, especially because the projects generally include some contact with people outside the educational program. Give the students ground rules for making outside contacts. For example, students doing a community assessment should have proper identification as students of your school to show to people they want to interview. They should have appropriate tools for data collection if they are asking people for information to assess health needs.

Supervising

A project may require indirect supervision by faculty. Schedule periodic meetings with the students to ascertain their progress and to monitor their performance. The supervisory meetings are also useful for teaching the processes involved in the project. For example, students doing a community study need instruction as they proceed through the steps involved, just as they do in learning how to take care of individuals in the hospital.

Appropriate supervision requires significant amounts of time. Under–graduate students need structure to meet the expectations of supervision. It is helpful simply to post a sign-up sheet with meeting times specified. This makes faculty availability to students apparent. If periodic meetings are required over the semester to discuss project work, designate the weeks in which the students must sign up. With students' busy schedules, e-mail may be an appropriate way to make appointments and also to discuss assignments. Part of a faculty member's role is determining when it is appropriate to make decisions or to introduce structure. With undergraduates, a lot of time is wasted unnecessarily by expecting the students to make decisions they have not learned how to make.

Grading

Projects may be time-consuming to grade. Some are best graded by observing students in the process of fulfilling the work, such as in doing health screening. Given the conditions under which such an event may occur, it is usually difficult to discriminate between various levels of performance. In such situations, other than to assess the safety of and respect for the client, evaluate the planning and overall implementation rather than specific interactions.

Other projects may require the production of a written work to be graded. As with papers such as those described previously, any written work is time-consuming to grade. Because the emphasis in assigning a project is on application, written materials should be graded with that in mind. In other words, there should be less emphasis on style and form unless that is indicated within the context of your course.

Presentations

Purpose

A presentation gives students the opportunity to share their work. It gives them the chance to organize information for an activity in a way more common for most nurses than written forms of presentation.

Preparation

Orienting students to a presentation is similar to giving guidelines for a paper. Tell them the parameters so that they can achieve the objectives. These issues are further discussed in the next major section. Some faculty members incorrectly see this format as an easy way to put on a course. Facilitating the experience of the students enrolled in a course is the responsibility of faculty. Be prepared to help correct misconceptions when students make mistakes in factual data and to help the entire group relate the material presented to the concepts of the course as a whole.

Grading

A presentation is fairly easy to grade if there is a checklist based on the criteria set in advance. It is best to grade at the time of the presentation.

TABLE 9.2   Checklist for Presentations

The following scale is used for the evaluation:

    5 Excellent

    4 Very good

    3 Average

    2 Below average

    1 Unsatisfactory

Content:

Meeting objectives	1	2	3	4	5
Accurate, current information	1	2	3	4	5
Appropriate coverage of information	1	2	3	4	5
Examples relating to content	1	2	3	4	5

Process:

Introduction	1	2	3	4	5
Organization	1	2	3	4	5
Quality of grammar, pronunciation	1	2	3	4	5
Summary	1	2	3	4	5

Scores Content _____	17–20 = A
Process _____	13–16 = B
Total _____	9–12 = C
Average _____	5–8 = D
	<5 = F

In some instances, there is value in having parts of the evaluation done by the other members of the class as well as by the faculty member and the presenter. If students are going to be evaluating each other and themselves, establish ground rules such as sticking to the criteria, using objective comments, describing specific behaviors, and using care in expressing negative opinions. A sample checklist is shown in Table 9.2.

Combinations of Assignments

Frequently, students are asked to combine two or three of the previously discussed forms of assignments. Whenever a second or third dimension is added to the assignment, you should take into consideration the extra work required along with the expectations for each dimension. Decide how much credit will be attached to each part while keeping in mind the basic objectives of the original assignment. If a project that takes a lot of time is involved, for example, most of the credit given should be attached to the portion requiring the most work. Some students may implement their projects well but do poorly in the class presentation. They should not be penalized on the presentation if the principal objectives were met by what the students did well.

TOOLS

Designing the Assignment

Description and Objectives

Start by describing the assignment in a brief, concise manner using straightforward language. It is important to have a clear purpose for the assignment. Next, list the objectives to be accomplished by the student in the completion of the assignment. A sample description and objectives are given in Table 9.3.

Required Content and Format

Although the description and objectives indicate the content, restate what is to be emphasized in the assignment. In the example given in Table 9.3, it may be helpful to stress that the focus is on two particular steps in the nursing process, although the student is to demonstrate some attention to the other two as well.

With undergraduates, supply them with a specific format to follow; for example, give them a specific outline. The outline or format can be useful for projects, papers, or presentations, and it helps to ensure that the students fulfill the requirements. A sample of a format is given in Table 9.4.

If appropriate, include format stipulations about the use of references. Designate the parameters in terms of how recent the references should be or what would be acceptable resources.

Grading the Assignment

Criteria for Evaluation

Base the criteria on the objectives and state them clearly. Specify in advance how the points will be assigned to each part of the assignment. Identifying such criteria gives the student information about the requirements

TABLE 9.3   An Assignment Description and Objectives

Nursing Care Study

The student will write a paper describing the nursing care of one patient. The paper will focus on the student's care only. All steps of the nursing process are to be discussed with emphasis on the planning and implementation steps. Prior to beginning the paper, the student must have the selected patient approved by the clinical instructor who will grade the paper.

Students are to meet the following objectives:

1. Summarize a data collection and identify significant data points for nursing intervention.
2. Demonstrate ability to set appropriate outcomes for the patient.
3. Identify the top three priorities in the patient's care.
4. Describe measurable criteria for evaluating outcomes.
5. Describe nursing interventions that relate to the identified priorities.
6. Use theoretical references to support nursing.
7. Devise at least one unique intervention.
8. Evaluate nursing-care outcomes using criteria.
9. Evaluate own performance of nursing care.
10. Use established standards for the preparation of a written paper.

for each portion of the assignment. Criteria help the student know the depth and breadth of information required for each section prior to undertaking the assignment. An example is given in Table 9.1 earlier in this chapter.

Submission Requirements

Clearly specify submission or completion requirements. When any written work is part of the assignment, encourage or require students to make a copy of their work before submitting the original for evaluation. With written work, set a submission date with some stipulation about how late submissions will be handled. If extensions are given without penalties for certain reasons, identify these exceptions. For example, illness or family emergencies may warrant an extension. Assess a reasonable penalty for late submissions based on the value of the assignment and the real inconvenience a late paper may cause. For example, assess a penalty of one to five points for each day the paper is late. Be sure to stipulate if weekends are

TABLE 9.4 Format for a Paper

Nursing Care Study

Format

Content

The study is to be in narrative form. Use the following major headings for the organization of the content.

Introduction: Describe the patient briefly.

Data Collection: Summarize the data collected on the patient and list the significant data on which your study will focus.

Outcome: State the outcome objectives you set.

Evaluation Criteria: Describe the criteria by which you planned to determine your success in meeting outcome objectives.

Priorities: List the top three priorities for care, and support your selection with references and data.

Interventions: Describe the interventions used for each objective, including references for their use. At least one intervention should be unique.

Evaluation: Using your evaluation criteria, describe how the patient met or did not meet those criteria. Evaluate your ability to perform the necessary nursing care using appropriate course objectives.

Summary: Summarize your role in the care of the patient.

or are not counted in the accumulation of days late. Give clear instructions regarding acceptable methods of submission of completed assignments; for example, make clear whether electronic submissions are acceptable.

If the assignment is a presentation, set the date for the presentation as far in advance as possible. Let the students know how much time will be available for the presentation so that they can plan accordingly. Make clear the criteria for evaluation of the presentation. Often, presentations are evaluated in terms of process as well as content. Establish clear ground rules about the relative weights of such grades and make the tool for the evaluation available to the students in advance. Have a plan in mind as to what to do with class time if the student or students scheduled to present are unable to do so.

If the assignment is a project, go over the requirements in detail with the students before they get started, and plan one or two meetings with the individuals or groups involved. Usually, students complete a project by submitting a written paper or by giving a presentation. This will make the submission criteria more complex. Bear in mind what the original purpose of the project was when evaluating the form in which it is reported.

INDIVIDUAL AND GROUP ASSIGNMENTS

Many assignments are made for individuals to complete. Because the kind of assignment being discussed here is often oriented toward synthesis and other high-level processes, evaluation of each person's ability to demonstrate these skills is important. Even if students may eventually use some of these skills as part of a team, there is benefit in each person's knowing something about each step in a process. Although this may result in a superficial treatment of some aspects of the assignment, at least each individual comes out of it with some knowledge about each part.

Individual assignments and individual evaluations are particularly appropriate in three situations, the first of which is when the assignment is something usually undertaken and accomplished by a single person in actual practice. The second circumstance is when an assignment is manageable for one person to complete in the amount of time you have allotted. The final situation is one in which it is important for each student to accomplish and demonstrate the skills involved.

Some major assignments are complex enough that group work is necessary to fulfill the requirements. For example, a community assessment is extremely complex if done thoroughly. For such an activity, students may learn more responsibility by focusing on a part of the assignment and sharing the responsibility.

For other assignments, a group effort may more closely simulate what happens in actual practice or convey a philosophical stance on how an activity should be carried out. A good example of this is a research proposal or project. Although a great deal of nursing research has been attempted by individuals, many expert nurse researchers emphasize the worth of nurses' doing more research in small teams. When projects are designed as group assignments, students see the value of such an approach.

Individual assignments by each person in the class are more time-consuming to grade than are a smaller number of group projects. With group projects, instead of grading 20 individual papers, you may have just six or eight group projects to grade.

Supervising and evaluating group work is more complex than working with individuals. Problems frequently occur as a result of difficulty within groups in working out individual responsibilities for the overall assignment. You can partially remedy this situation by meeting with the groups and helping them to establish their own ground rules. After all, if part of the intent is for them to learn how to work in a group, students need guidance on this as well as in dealing with the content itself. Before making the assignment a group activity, give some thought to how the groups can present their final product so that assessment of individual achievement is possible.

Decide how to handle grievances over allegations by group members that others in the group are not taking their share of responsibility. For example, if one person seems not to be doing his or her work, what proof would you require of this? How would you deal with it if it were proved to you? Getting caught in the middle of this kind of situation is pretty uncomfortable, especially if you are not prepared.

Support all the students and help them to establish some ground rules for dealing with the identified problem. Often the students who originally complained are as much at fault as is the one about whom they are complaining.

One way to avoid this type of situation is to have frequent meetings with the groups. The students' ability to work as a group in such meetings will reflect how they are doing when the group works alone. The supervision of group work is discussed in more detail in chapter 4.

FINAL WORDS

Major assignments help instructors evaluate students' abilities to accomplish high-level objectives. To ensure a successful outcome, spend time in the design of the assignment requirements and criteria for evaluation. As with other teaching tools, putting effort in the design of assignments will make the assignments more manageable for you to evaluate.

10

Designing and Grading a Minor Assignment

A minor assignment is different from a major assignment in that it is less substantive in terms of depth and breadth of content involved, time required for completion, and the amount of credit attached to the finished product. Some assignments considered major in one context may be minor in another. For example, a critique of a research article would be a major assignment for students initially learning about research. For graduate students, such a critique would be minor. However, other minor assignments are fairly typical and may be given that designation whether in an undergraduate or a graduate course.

Generally, minor assignments are focused on something specific, such as a short essay about a student's thoughts on an event or concept. Such assignments should take only an hour or two to complete. The credit given for minor assignments is relatively small compared with the credit for other course requirements that call for more work. In some instances, credit may be given in a blanket manner, such as when there is a requirement for four short essays, and the student receives a predetermined amount of credit as long as the essays are submitted at the specified times. The faculty member does not have to evaluate the quality of each essay, only note that each was submitted.

GOALS

Minor assignments are used to measure medium- to higher-level objectives. As with major assignments, certain tools help in the evaluation of learning that is not easily measured by objective means.

TYPES OF MINOR ASSIGNMENTS

Short Essay

A short essay is approximately two to five typed pages long. The content is focused on one objective or one incident. For example, such a paper may describe a student's first reaction to a given clinical setting. There are few or no references required, with emphasis being placed on the student's ideas or involvement. The format is simple, perhaps including only an introduction, the body of the paper with no subtopics, and a conclusion.

Journal Entry

A journal entry is very short and may be completed in one page. It is focused very specifically and briefly and describes the student's position or ideas relating to an objective or event. Such an assignment could be used to allow the student to describe feelings about a particular topic or experience. Table 10.1 shows a sample journal entry.

Critique

A critique is a critical discussion. In nursing education, a critique is often done on the elements of a published research study. A critique helps to

TABLE 10.1   A Journal Entry

My Most Challenging Patient

My most challenging patient was a 23-year-old woman who was admitted with acute abdominal pain, diarrhea, and projectile vomiting. I had to start an IV, insert an NG tube, and give her an injection in preparation to go to surgery. It took at least 24 minutes to talk her into each procedure while she whined and verbally abused me for trying to do each thing.

The last thing I did before she went to the OR was to help her with the bedpan. While I was cleaning it, she said, "I think you became a nurse just to make people suffer." I said, "I can see why you might feel that way, but I really want to help you." She said, "Ha!" I made sure the bed rails were secure and left.

When the aide came with the carrier to take her to the OR, I went to help transfer her. When they started to wheel her away, she said, "I am so scared." I took her hand and said, "I will go with you." I held her hand until they took her into the OR. The last thing she said to me was, "Thanks, nurse." I felt wonderful!

foster a student's appreciation of the parts of research. By using established criteria to evaluate a research study, a student learns to use critical thinking skills.

Students need guidelines to learn to perform critiques. Most texts on nursing research provide useful outlines to give students the necessary structure. In an undergraduate research course, a critique may itself be a major assignment and may be done over many weeks as the students learn more about the research process. However, as a student advances, the process of doing critiques becomes just a part of more major assignments.

Students are evaluated on their ability to apply the relevant criteria correctly and to draw the appropriate kinds of conclusions. For students who are just learning about the process, requirements are less stringent. For more advanced students, it would be appropriate to expect them to recognize subtleties or sophisticated aspects of the process involved in doing the critique.

Response Paper

A response paper has the purpose of asking students to respond to something in particular, usually a journal article. This assignment permits students to demonstrate critical thinking and encourages them to synthesize what they are reading. Students may be asked to identify applications of an article that is primarily theoretical, for example.

As with other assignments, set more specific guidelines for students in undergraduate courses. If you are working with graduate students, the assignment may be open-ended, and part of the expectation would be for them to identify their own focus for such an activity.

Brief Presentation

The brief presentation is different from the presentation discussed as a major assignment because it requires little preparation outside of class and is very specific in focus, such as the written assignments discussed earlier in this chapter. For example, students may be expected to present their work with their assigned patients in a clinical conference.

Brief presentations give students the opportunity to practice expressing and sometimes defending their ideas in an open forum. Give students guidelines about what they are expected to present, and provide the group with ground rules on how to behave in such a forum. As with other minor assignments, evaluation may be more a function of giving credit to the student for simply completing the presentation, rather than trying to evaluate it in the way one would a major presentation.

Debates

Assign students or ask them to volunteer to argue for or against a proposition. Require them to work in teams or as individuals to develop their arguments. Specify in advance how long the students will have to present their sides as well as the time permitted for rebuttal. Following the debate, the rest of the class can respond to the strength and validity of the arguments. As with other assignments, be explicit about all the parameters involved, such as time, resources used, clarity of presentation, and so on, just as with other presentations.

Logs

A log may be kept on a weekly basis to deal with the interpersonal aspects of some clinical experiences. Logs are probably more common assignments in psychiatric settings or nursing experiences in community health. A log helps students to evaluate and incorporate their personal experiences in a situation uncommon to their usual activities.

Give students structure as to what content and process are expected in the log. For example, ask them to take no more than one or two notebook pages for each entry. In each entry, ask them to describe the most interesting thing that happened during the week, or ask them to discuss how a particular concept was applied or how a certain objective was met.

Rather than grading the logs, you may give the students credit simply for completing and submitting the logs as required. This approach is especially important if you are asking students to be honest and open about their own feelings—they should be given credit for doing so, but you can hardly grade feelings. It would be more appropriate to give encouraging comments, such as "You really opened up this week" or "This must have been tough for you." If the entry pertains to something factual or cognitive, you might say, "You did a good job of describing this situation" or "This is a good example of the concept."

TOOLS

Designing the Assignment

Start with a concise description of the assignment and the objectives to be met. Describe the expected format and the content to be included. Give the students a sample of what is required in the assignment or guidelines to follow. Minor assignments are always done on an individual basis. These assignments are oriented to individual activities, such as reading or analysis and synthesis of a personal experience.

Grading the Assignment

In the case of minor assignments, students are frequently given credit just for completing the assignment according to expectations and submitting it at the proper time. If planning to grade a minor assignment, be clear about the criteria and keep them reasonable in accord with the extent of the work required. Specify the requirements for submission or completion. If multiple parts of a minor assignment are required, such as short essays, specify the intervals at which they are to be submitted.

Minor assignments take little time to grade but may still be time-consuming overall, especially if multiple-part assignments are required several times during a term. Students' submitted written work should be evaluated by some method such as a brief written comment. If finding time to evaluate students' work is a problem, then decrease the requirements and expectations. Evaluating students' work is an important task, and adequate time must be assigned to read and evaluate student submissions. It is common for new instructors to assign too much work the first time they teach a course. Talk to colleagues who have taught the same course or similar courses to find out about the amount of work students can handle and about how to evaluate their abilities reasonably.

FINAL WORDS

Minor assignments can help instructors evaluate skills that are difficult to test by objective means. They permit the students to demonstrate specific abilities in a brief format.

FURTHER READING

McKeachie, W. J. (2002). *Teaching tips: Strategies, research, and theory for college university teachers.* (11th ed.). Boston: Houghton Mifflin.

11

Test Construction and Analysis

Tests are an inevitable part of teaching. After you have taught a class, tests are a way to evaluate the students' grasp of the material as well as a way to assess your success at conveying the material. It is important to think of testing in this two-dimensional manner: the better the test, the better the evaluation of both the students and faculty.

Before planning a test, determine whether it is the most appropriate evaluation tool. Why give a test? If the objectives to be evaluated relate to the lower cognitive levels (knowledge, comprehension, and application), a paper-and-pencil test may be the most efficient way to find out if the students learned the content of the class. If the objectives pertain to psychomotor skills, the best way to evaluate is to observe the students perform the skills. Some students may be able to describe all the steps of a skill in the right order but may not be at all able to demonstrate the skill correctly or safely. On the other hand, some students may have difficulty in describing the skill, but may be able to demonstrate it well and safely.

For higher-level cognitive objectives or objectives in the affective domain, it is difficult to write test items, especially for an objective test. Other types of assignments, such as those described in chapters 9 and 10, often may better measure such objectives.

GOALS

The primary goal of testing is to evaluate the ability of students to achieve the desired outcomes as described by course objectives. Secondarily, testing students may help in evaluating the teacher's effectiveness in helping the students to achieve the desired outcomes.

CONTEXT OF TESTING

Before beginning use of testing tools, consider the context in which tests are used. Part of planning a course is determining how much testing is needed to assess the students' achievement of course objectives. If the course content is complex and extensive, more tests are required. An example would be a course with advanced theory and practical applications, such as a senior-year course. In courses in which the content is abstract and other assignments determine part of the course grade, there will be fewer tests. For example, fewer tests are needed in a course focusing on trends and issues. In such a course, subjective assignments such as papers or presentations are more suitable.

Frequency of Tests

Tests should be proctored at reasonable intervals during a course to allow sufficient time for the students to learn the content. If there are several small tests and a final examination, each small test should cover the same amount of content, have about the same number of items, and be given at regular intervals.

Weighting Tests

The value of each test in determining the course grade should be based on the amount of content each one covers. All tests of a similar nature, such as unit tests, should be given the same weight unless there is a difference in the amount of content covered. Unless earlier tests given in the course are shorter tests or cover less important material, they should be considered equally with later tests. The exception would be for comprehensive examinations, such as a final exam, which would probably be longer and therefore would be given more weight. An example of the master plan for giving tests in a course is discussed in the subsequent section on test plans.

TOOLS

Test Plans

A test plan is sometimes called a "test blueprint." As both names suggest, these are tools that help in planning the content for tests.

Course Test Plan

Before developing individual test plans, develop a master plan for all the tests in the course. For example, if the course is fairly complex, you may decide to have three unit tests plus a comprehensive final examination. Table 11.1 shows a course test plan for such a situation.

In preparing a course test plan, take into account such factors as lecture periods in which little actual content may be conveyed, such as the first day of class when a lot of time is spent discussing the orientation to the course. Other such periods to consider could include spring break or holidays that preempt course time. Finally, it is a good idea to avoid giving a test in the last week of classes, in order to help students begin to get ready for final exams. Some schools have policies that require that the last class week be free of tests. Overall, try to come up with a balance so that each test will be over the same amount of content, and each content area can be adequately tested. For the final examination in the situation illustrated in Table 11.1, a larger number of items for the content from the last week of class is appropriate because the students in this example have not been previously tested on that material. This portion would include the same number of items as there were on the unit tests, as well as additional items that equal the number of items covering each section for the comprehensive part of the final exam.

Individual Test Plan

Although there is a fairly standard way to produce a grid for a test plan, each teacher has to decide what will constitute the parameters. The parameters depend on the type of course and the thrust of the course. For example, a simple plan may have the lectures on one axis and the parts of the nursing process on the other. Such a plan with equal weightings for each cell is set up in Table 11.2.

TABLE 11.1   A Course Test Plan

Date	Test	Content	Items	Weight (%)
2/15	Unit 1	Weeks 1–5	60	20
3/21	Unit 2	Weeks 6–10	60	20
4/20	Unit 3	Weeks 11–15	60	20
5/2	Final	Weeks 16 + Comprehensive	120	40

TABLE 11.2 A Test Plan Without Differential Weightings for Cells

	Assess	Plan	Implement	Evaluate	Total
Lec. 1	3	3	3	3	12
Lec. 2	3	3	3	3	12
Lec. 3	3	3	3	3	12
Lec. 4	3	3	3	3	12
Totals	12	12	12	12	48

The sample test plan in Table 11.2 shows the lecture numbers on the vertical axis. For clarity, an abbreviated version of the lecture title, such as "Immobility" or "ADL," could be listed in each space. The horizontal axis indicates the parts of the nursing process with a final column heading for row totals.

The grid in Table 11.2 was constructed by simply multiplying the number of columns by the number of rows. This gives the number of cells (16). Presume that 60 minutes were available for the testing period. The students were given about 1 minute per item, and the time available was divided by the number of cells (60 ÷ 16 = 3.75). In Table 11.2, each cell has a 3 in it. It was decided to have the same number of items for each cell, and the number had to be a round number; if the result (3.75) had been rounded up to 4, then 4 would have been multiplied by the number of cells to get the total items for the test (4 × 16). 64 items would have been required, which would have been pushing some students to respond in 60 minutes. However, rounding the number down to 3 resulted in a requirement of a total of 48 items. Table 11.3 summarizes these steps.

The plan in Table 11.2 was based on the assumption that the content to be tested in each cell was equally as important as the content in every other cell. As a matter of fact, though, it is possible and perhaps important to put greater weight on some aspects than on others. The sample plan shown in Table 11.4 reflects a situation in which judgments have been made about the differential weighting of content.

In developing the sample plan in Table 11.4, the first step is to determine the number of items in each cell of the plan by deciding on priorities about the most important content covered by the plan. The first question to ask is, How should each component of the horizontal axis be weighted? In the

TABLE 11.3   Calculating Number of Items per Cell When Weightings Are Equal

Step 1: Rows × columns = number of cells

Step 2: Time for test ÷ number of cells = items per cell

Step 3: If items per cell is not a round number, round it up or
down so that the items per cell × number of cells ≤ time for test

TABLE 11.4   A Test Plan Based on Lecture Content and Parts of the Nursing Process With Differential Weighting of Content[a]

	Assess	Plan	Implement	Evaluate	Total
Lec. 1	2.75/3	2.75/3	3.67/4	1.83/2	11/12
Lec. 2	2.75/2	2.75/2	3.67/4	1.83/2	11/10
Lec. 3	2.75/3	2.75/2	3.67/4	1.83/2	11/11
Lec. 4	2.75/2	2.75/3	3.67/4	1.83/2	11/11
Lec. 5	2/2	2/2	3.67/3	1.33/0	8/7
Lec. 6	2/3	2/2	2.67/3	1.33/1	8/9
Totals	15/15	15/14	20/22	10/9	60/60

[a]The projected number of items for each cell is shown in italics. The number on the right side of the slash in each cell represents the actual number planned for the test.

sample plan, the "implementation" step of the nursing process is weighted more heavily than the other steps. About a third of the resultant test would be on that step. The assessment and planning phases are weighted equally with one another. The evaluation step has fewer items because the class is an early course in which students might be expected to have little skill in the evaluation aspect.

The next question is, How should the content on the vertical axis be weighted? In the sample in Table 11.4, the content in the first four lectures is of equal importance. However, the last two lectures are not given as much weight. Perhaps in this sample situation, the first four lectures cover complex content that might require more items to sample the students' knowledge adequately. The last lectures might be as long, but they would include less complex content or content that could be tested more easily with fewer questions.

The test being planned in Table 11.4 would be given in a 60-minute period, which gives the grand total for the number of items. The decisions about the axes lead to the assignment of hypothetical totals for each row and column. To calculate the number of items that would fit into each cell, the column and row totals for that cell are multiplied and then divided by the total number of items. For example, for the cell under "Assessment" for the first lecture, 15 multiplied by 11 and divided by 60 makes 2.75.

In order to arrive at the actual numbers for each cell in Table 11.4, round the fractional numbers up or down. To determine which direction to go, consider what content is being tested within each cell. For each lecture look at each lecture objective and see what is emphasized. For the first lecture, the first three steps in the nursing process are about equally emphasized in the objectives and content and should have the maximum number of items to sample the students' knowledge. However, it may be that those two items would be sufficient to indicate if a student could adequately evaluate the success of the earlier steps in dealing with the topic.

For every decision to round a projected number up or down, a number in another cell had to be rounded in the opposite direction so that the final total of items is correct. In the previous hypothetical test, it was decided that two items were sufficient for testing both assessment and planning for the second lecture. These numbers were then rounded down to accommodate those that were increased. In one column where all the numbers were rounded up, the new total was higher than the projected total. Because this column was to be weighted heavily, then lower totals were accepted in two other columns.

Another factor to note is that one cell is empty. Sometimes the content may not lend itself to any items in a given cell, or it might be expected that the students will not be able to answer items about it because there is not a relevant lecture objective pertaining to that knowledge. This example that has been discussed shows that even though there is a technical way to calculate the item totals, professional judgment should be used to determine the final number of items for each cell.

Some situations call for only one item, whereas others require more than one to test an objective. An objective on the cognitive level of knowledge would be, "Define pertussis." One item could sufficiently determine if students could do this. Higher-level objectives would require not only more complex items, but also more items. For example, "Develop an evaluation plan for the care of a child with leukemia" may require several objective items or one short answer item worth several points.

Although in the example the values in the cells of the test plan have been referred to as equivalent to numbers of items, one could think of these as numbers of points. For example, in the evaluation cell for Lecture No. 1, there could be two multiple-choice items worth one point each or one short answer item worth two points.

Test-Item Bank

Database programs, such as Microsoft Access, can manage a bank of test items. These programs allow categorization and filing of items with a variety of descriptors so that a set of test items that meet certain criteria can be reviewed. For example, all the items on nursing interventions for a depressed patient can be selected. Then from the items available, the number required for the test plan can be selected. These programs also allow the computer to select the number of items required from those stored.

One feature in the marketing of many nursing texts today is the inclusion of a test-item bank on computer disks. These items are based directly on the content in the respective texts, of course, but it is usually possible to edit the items as well as add new items to the bank. Other texts have a companion instructor manual that contains test items for the purpose of supplementing your personal bank. These are good sources because the items are already categorized and referenced to the text. Although the instructor may still wish to produce test items, these sources can help to give more variety and provide many questions to each content area. Some publishers provide online instructors' guides for the textbooks with test items related to each chapter.

Proficiency Examinations

Many schools have provisions for students to challenge courses. This means the student may earn credit other than by enrolling in a course. One way this may be done is by a teacher-made proficiency examination. A proficiency exam should be based on the same fundamental elements as the course. Examinees should be required to show that they know at least as much as the average student who took the course and passed it.

For a course in which tests are the only means for arriving at grades for students, test plans can be used in determining the number of items and weightings so that the content is tested similarly. Use the same items or similar items as on regular tests in the course. Some faculty members use a recent final exam for this purpose if the exam is comprehensive.

If part of the course grade is determined by means other than tests, the process to challenge should include the same means. For example, if the course has a practical component such as doing a physical assessment or demonstrating other psychomotor skills, a portion of the exam should replicate that aspect. In a beginning research course, students may have to pass written exams and critique a research report. The same performance would be expected of those who challenge the course.

NUTS AND BOLTS

Types of Items

Objective

The most common items are objective items. The objectivity involved means that there is one objectively determined correct answer. The students must choose from answers provided. Examples are multiple-choice, true-or-false, and matching questions. Anyone educated in the United States has probably been exposed to all of these, but each kind is described briefly here.

Multiple-choice items include a stem that describes a person or situation and asks a question about it. The student must select the correct answer from a set of options. True-or-false items are usually one-sentence statements. The student must decide whether the statement is true or false. Matching items include two lists of terms. The student is asked to match terms from one list with terms on the other list according to some specification. Objective items are easy to grade because a test key permits rapid marking or because a computer or scanner can grade them.

Subjective

The subjectivity involved in subjective items is that of the person grading the items. The student is given some latitude in answering, and the teacher determines if the answer is correct. The student must provide an answer without any cues. The basic types are short-answer items and essay questions.

In short-answer items, the student must recall the correct information without the prompting of options. These items call for a few words or at most a sentence or two. These are close to objective items because there is usually only one correct response. An essay question requires a lengthy response and calls for the student to demonstrate more than recall of facts. The student may be expected to demonstrate high-level cognitive objectives, such as analysis or synthesis. Essay items may be used to test students' ability to meet objectives in the affective domain.

Subjective items take longer to grade. With short-answer items, it takes a little longer to recognize a word or phrase while scanning the answer sheet than it does to simply recognize if the correct letter of the right option has been filled in. With lengthy answers, even more time is required to read and evaluate the students' responses.

Writing Test Items

A good test item should meet the following criteria: (1) it relates to important content that the students should retain, (2) it is unambiguous, and (3) if it is an objective item, it has one and only one correct answer among the choices provided. In addition to these criteria, there are several other important principles to consider in writing test items. The majority of the principles pertain to objective items, but also included are some that would pertain to either type of item as well as principles specifically for subjective items.

1. *Significance of content.* If asking the students to respond to an item on a test, you should ask yourself if it is really important for them to know the specific piece of information they are being asked about. It would be easy to ask for something specific like, "When are immunizations for pertussis, rubella, polio, and tetanus given in the first year of a child's life?" The options could be a laundry list of time intervals. Is this information they should memorize? How long will they retain it even if they do? It may be more valuable to ask a question such as, "What would be the most effective way to help a mother of a small child to remember when to get her child's immunizations?" This is a higher-level question, and it also tests for application that would be transferable to other nursing situations.

Frequently in baccalaureate programs, faculty test over the more complex content common in the program and may never ask simple questions on basic nursing practice. Baccalaureate graduates may be able to answer questions on metabolism at the cellular level, and yet not be able to recognize a diet high in vitamin C. The critical question is this: what will the graduates need to know to be safe, competent beginning practitioners at their level of preparation?

2. *Clarity.* The item should be easy to read, so that the students spend their time thinking about the correct answer rather than trying to decipher the meaning of the question. Use vocabulary that is common to what the students read for the course. Use simple terms they are likely to know, unless recognizing the terminology is part of what you are testing. Do not use abbreviations of terms unless the term is spelled out initially followed by the abbreviation in parentheses.

Make sure that your stem and your options are as unambiguous as possible. An example of an ambiguous stem would be "Mr. Warren is receiving Prozac. One morning he asks his nurse the name of the drug. She tells him it is to help his mood. What is this called?" Once the student reads the options, the stem may seem less ambiguous, but initially, it is probably not clear what the word *this* refers to. Does it mean the reason for the patient's question or does it refer to the nurse's response? A less ambiguous question would be "What would the nurse's response be called?"

3. *One correct answer.* The correct answer may not be comprehensive, but what there is of it should be correct and should answer the question in the stem. For example, in response to the question, "Which of the following is a reason people experience crisis?" a correct answer would be "Lack of a support system." There are other correct answers that contribute, but this is a correct answer even by itself. None of the other options should be true. If there could be several correct answers but one is more important or more significant, the others can be used as distracters but the stem must make clear that the students are to choose the most significant factor from the options.

4. *Clear basis for a correct response.* The criterion for what the student must choose as the correct response should be clearly indicated. For example, what would be the correct response to the following sample item?

Mr. Carson complains at length about pains in his feet and back. No pathology has been discovered to account for this pain, and the staff believes this complaining is a symptom of low self-esteem and need for attention. When Mr. Carson begins complaining to you, what would you say?

a. "You are just seeking attention."
b. "I will sit and talk with you for a while."
c. "If you quit talking about the pain, it will go away."
d. "I will come back when you feel better."

Even though option "b" is the most therapeutic choice, because the stem asked the student "What would you say?" any answer could be correct. Specify the criterion by which the right answer is to be determined, using such phrases as "the best thing to say (or do)," "the first thing," "the highest priority," "the most helpful." The person who is taking action should be the nurse or the student assuming the role of the nurse. Then ask, "What should the nurse say?"

5. *Believable distracters.* Each incorrect option should be somewhat believable, so that at least a few students would choose each one. Good distracters are things that the "average" person might think or things that are common misconceptions. The following item helps to illustrate this.

What is the first priority in dealing with a psychotic patient?

a. Decrease his hallucinations
b. Promote his developing trust
c. Improve his self-esteem
d. Increase his interactions with others

An intelligent person who has not been studying psychiatric nursing lately would be likely to think that the most important thing in working with someone who is psychotic is to deal with the most obvious evidence of psychosis—hallucinations. Others may guess that such people should interact with other people to help them become less withdrawn. Others who do not really understand working with such patients may think you should focus on low self-esteem, which they consider part of the psychotic person's problems. The student who understands the fundamental aspects of working with these patients will know that trust is essential to accomplish any of the other goals.

6. *Length.* Each multiple-choice item should take about 1 minute to read and answer. If you want to provide a hypothetical patient to whom the students will refer, include only the data that will apply to the items. The exception to this would be when it is important for the students to

demonstrate they can discriminate between extraneous and important data. Look at the following item and see how much could be deleted while keeping the question as a good item.

Mary Jones is a 23-year-old married woman with a high school education. She works as a secretary for an oil company. She has been diagnosed as having rheumatoid arthritis. Which of the following would be the most appropriate set of instructions for maintaining her joint mobility?

   a. Take aspirin only once a day, and apply heat to joints.
   b. Exercise moderately, and protect joints from exposure to cold air.
   c. Eat plenty of green vegetables, and take extra iron.
   d. Maintain internal rotation of joints, and drink extra fluids.

Unless planning to have several items pertaining to "Mary Jones," the majority of the information in the stem is irrelevant because selecting the correct answer is not dependent on any of the information specific to the patient. The stem can be cut down to the following: "In order to maintain joint mobility in a person with rheumatoid arthritis, which of the following would be the most appropriate set of instructions?"

7. *Simple multiple-choice.* The current preference among many nursing educators is for simple multiple-choice items rather than multiple-multiple-choice. A simple multiple-choice item allows specific evaluation of the student knowledge in that content area. In a multiple-multiple-choice item, a student may choose the correct option by eliminating one of the sub-options, without understanding the reason for the correct answer. Another benefit of simple multiple-choice items is that these prepare the students for the RN licensing examination. This exam is made up entirely of simple multiple-choice items.

8. *Distribution of correct answers.* Keep track of the letters or numbers of the correct options for items written. Over the test as a whole, each option should be the correct answer about the same number of times. Keep a tally as items are written for a test. If using some previously written items, note the correct options to start with so that the equal numbers can be maintained. This helps to prevent students from answering correctly just because they may have noticed a tendency to have the third option as the

correct one a lot of the time. To avoid this problem completely, alphabetize the options in descending order. If the subsequent option begins with the same word, go to the next word to sort in alphabetical order.

9. *Options with numbers.* When using options with numbers, each option should be exclusive. For example:

What is the acceptable dosage of diazepam (Valium) for treatment of anxiety?

  a. 2 mg b.i.d.
  b. 4–40 mg daily
  c. 20–40 mg daily
  d. up to 50 mg

Yikes! Where is the student to start in sorting this one out? The second option is correct in terms of being the range of acceptable doses, but 20 to 40 mg is included within that range. The first option is correct as a daily dose even though it does not reflect a range. The fourth option is the only one that is clearly unacceptable.

Numbers should make sense for the situation being described. Values that are too small or too large are unlikely to be chosen. They should also be in the same type of measurement, such as all in milligrams or all in ounces, unless part of what the item is testing is the ability of the student to convert from one system of measurement to another. It is usually best to present numbers in increments from small to large.

10. *Cues to the right answer.* Be careful to avoid echoing words from the stem in the correct option. The following example shows this error.

What process do nurses use in caring for patients?

  a. Problem solving
  b. Scientific approach
  c. Nursing process
  d. Analysis

Another inadvertent clue would be to use a plural reference in the stem when only the correct option contains a plural noun.

Which people are at highest risk for committing suicide?

a. Teenagers
b. A professional
c. An old person
d. A woman

Avoid direct quotes in options unless all of the options sound the same.

What is the definition of "ethnocentrism?"

a. Thinking your culture is the center of the universe
b. Having a God-oriented belief system
c. The belief that one's own cultural or social group is superior to others
d. Failing to take culture into account in working with patients

The third option sounds like a textbook definition of a term whereas the incorrect options begin with a gerund and do not sound as formal. This could be corrected by restating the other options in parallel language, such as in the statements below:

• The idea that one's culture is the center of the universe
• The presence of a belief system that is God-oriented
• The tendency to exclude cultural concerns from interactions

11. *"None of the above" and "All of the above."* If you use options like "None of the above" or "All of the above," there are some things to keep in mind.

• Sometimes include these options when they are wrong as well as when they are the correct ones.
• When including "None of the above," indicate in the stem that the student may expect this option. For example, "Which of the following, if any, would be the right breathing technique for a woman in the first stage of labor?"
• Do not overuse "All of the above" just because it may be difficult to come up with three good distracters for each item. This makes the test much easier than if the students had to make real discriminations.

12. *Using negatives.* Stems that ask students questions couched in negative terms are more difficult to read and may inadvertently trick the students. If using a negative term or if asking for the reverse of what is usually asked, emphasize it in some way to draw the students' attention. Some examples are "Which of the following would not be an appropriate toy for a four-year-old child in the hospital?" or "What would be the least effective treatment for a strained muscle?"

Be careful about introducing double negatives, which may confound the students' understanding. For example:

Stem: When would you not suggest a patient cough and deep breathe after surgery?
Option: When he is not receiving artificial ventilation.

13. *Stereotyped or sexist language.* Take as much care to respect the rights and feelings of students when writing test items as when interacting with them in person. The following are some problems encountered by nursing faculty when writing test items.

- Attributing unintelligent or negative qualities to hypothetical patients or nurses who are in particular ethnic or gender groups. "Maria Gomez is a poorly educated woman with a history of child abuse." It is appropriate that some items on your test should have different ethnic groups represented, but be sure that they are not included only in such negative contexts.
- Attaching names that have usually been used with unflattering connotations for certain ethnic groups. "Jemimah is a black woman who does not understand conception control."
- Implying that one gender is not as bright or as good as the other. "Paul is a straight A student, whereas Mary is barely passing."
- Implying that patients of one gender are only interested in stereotyped activities or involved in certain roles. An example of this would be leaving the father out when discussing hypothetical situations relating to children.
- Neglecting to use male names for any of the hypothetical nurses in your test items and making all the nurses women and most of the patients men (unless you are dealing with obstetrics).

- Using certain ethnic groups' names when describing aggressive or other behaviors that may have negative connotations.

To avoid these pitfalls, do not make everyone a Smith, Jones, or Garcia. Try to use typical sounding names from a variety that have different ethnic origins. If comparing two people, one of who has a negative attribution, make both the people of the same gender and same ethnic group. However, it is best to avoid using names altogether and to use neutral terms such as patient, client, or nurse. In this way no one will be offended by the test items.

14. *Introduce humor with care.* Some faculty members like to include one or two items intended to be funny for the purpose of relieving tension. Ironically, this maneuver sometimes has the opposite effect. If the attempt is ambiguous or if the students are so engrossed in the testing process that they overlook the intent, they may become distracted. If an item is meant to be funny, either make it the last item or tag it clearly as such.

15. *Specify response length.* When writing short-answer or essay questions, indicate how much of a response is expected. For example, with a short answer item, provide a blank to fill in that limits the length of the response. Make sure the blank is of sufficient length to accommodate the expected response. An example would be: "What is the average age at which infants' teeth first emerge? ____months"

For essay questions, specify the length, and also make any other applicable parameters clear. The following two examples show this.

Example 1: Using 100 to 125 words, identify and discuss one of the major contributions Florence Nightingale made to the foundation of modern nursing. Describe the impact of her innovation on nursing as it was practiced in her era.

Example 2: Select a situation with ethical implications from the following: abortion, total life support, sterilization, death and dying, in vitro fertilization. State your position and analyze how you arrived at your position using either a deontological or a teleological model. Your response should be around 250 words.

Assembling a Test

There are some technical aspects to putting the test together that make the test look polished and ensure the students will not be at a disadvantage because of extraneous factors that have nothing to do with their knowledge.

Order

When assembling a test, put the items in the same order as the content was presented in class. This means that all items over one part of the content are together. It also means that they are in order from the less difficult to the more difficult within each group, because that is the usual way content is presented.

Arrangement

The beginning and ending of the components of each item should be clear. All the parts of an item should be on the same page. For example, do not have the stem on one page and the options or part of the options on another. All items should be presented in a standard format. The examples given earlier in this chapter show a standard format.

Options

In a multiple-choice item, the options should always be listed in the same way, such as vertically, not in a horizontal list. List every set of options either flush with the left margin or aligned along an indent of the same number of spaces each time.

Each item should have the same number of options. Write four options for each item. It is difficult to come up with four distracters for each item, as is needed if there are five options for each item. Three options are too few because this increases the possibility of students' getting the correct answer by chance. Another reason to use the same number of options for each item is to avoid causing the student to make a mistake such as marking "d" when they mean to choose the last option, which might be "e."

Proofing

Always proofread your own tests. Even the best typists make errors. Make sure that each item is complete and that they are all arranged in the chosen format. Check for misspellings or missing words. Be especially alert for negative words such as "no" and "not" that may have been omitted.

Grading Tests

There is often no need to hand-grade multiple-choice items given that many people rely on machines. If grading tests by hand, do everything possible in advance to simplify the procedure. This would include having answer sheets separate from the test itself. Set them up so that the scoring key can easily be aligned with the answers for ease in reading and marking. If giving subjective tests that have to be hand-graded, plan ahead of time to allow for the time needed to grade the papers. Often teaching assistants can be valuable in assisting with grading subjective tests

Test Analysis

Most educational institutions have centralized computer services to calculate test reliability and item analysis. The usual data provided is an alphabetical listing of the students with their individual raw score, percentage score, and percentage rank. Also included is the number of students, number of items on the test, maximum possible score, mean score, mean percentage score, standard deviation, and a frequency distribution of scores. For teacher-made tests, reliabilities between 0.60 and 0.80 are considered good. Anything less than 0.60 should raise a red flag. The reliability of a test can be increased by making it longer. Even though it seems difficult to write more items on an area of content, there are many possible items that could be asked about any subject. If asking a dozen questions about proper ways to position an immobilized patient, a student who really understands the principles should be able to get most of the questions right. However, even a good student could miss two of twelve items on the subject. What if only two questions were asked and those two were the ones the student did not know? On the other hand, a weak student may answer only half the items on positioning, but one of the six could be one of the two the other student answered incorrectly. This would give a different picture of the students' knowledge. Therefore, the more items, the better the indication you get of the strengths and weaknesses of your students. If it is possible to add some items, especially on a complex area of content, even a little may help to make your results more reliable.

Item Analysis

Item analysis is used to help determine the content validity of the test. Did the test measure what it was supposed to measure?

Information provided by an item analysis helps to improve items before they are used again. It also quickly reveals that there was clearly no correct answer or the wrong answer was keyed as correct. The item analysis will tell the number of students who responded to each option. It will also indicate the difficulty of the item. Depending on how the data is presented, an easy question is determined on the basis that nearly everyone answered it correctly. When there are questions that a high number of students have missed, examine them to be sure they are fair. Maybe a lot of students missed them because they were not well written; or the material may not have been covered well enough for them to have understood the important points. On the other hand, when the correlation between a given item and the whole test is examined, it may be concluded that the item is a good discriminator between the better and the weaker students. This will be discussed further later on.

Evaluating Distractors

By looking at the percentages of students who chose incorrect options, one can more easily evaluate how well the distractors are working. If no one ever selects a certain distractor after an item is used two or three times, there is no point in having it there. Try a new distractor or try rewriting it to make the item more challenging. If one distractor gets chosen about as often as the correct option, this may give an indication of areas of content that are difficult for students to understand. This information is beneficial when planning the content and teaching methods for the next class.

Discrimination

Sometimes the correlation value between the item and the test is referred to as the discrimination power because it shows how well the item helps to discriminate between the students who do well on the test and those who do not.

The discrimination power is a helpful statistic. A statistically significant value indicates that the particular item is doing a good job of differentiating between the students' performance on the test. These items help to identify who should be in the various groups for grades. However, if too many of the items have high discrimination power, the test may be too difficult for the group you are testing.

Because this is a correlation statistic, the values range from -1.0 to $+1.0$. Items with values around 0 to 0.30 are usually not discriminating. Items with negative values are negatively correlated with the test as a whole. This is fairly unusual—especially to see a negative correlation that is significant. This result means that students who do well on the test are tending to miss the item. This could be because there is some room for interpretation and the better students read more into the question or understand the information better.

Revising Items

The data from the statistics will help with improving the items. Some of the ways in which this helps have already been mentioned. When first reviewing the statistics, make notes about obvious problems. However, often it is better to allow some time before working on revisions because revising too quickly may result in rewriting much better test items. Time will give objectivity when evaluating these items.

Have other faculty members review the items. Even if the content is not their area of expertise, they can identify process strengths and weaknesses in the items. Because they do not necessarily know the content, they can sometimes pick out ways in which the correct answer is cued by the stem. If items are ambiguous, they can tell because they do not know the content to the degree the item writers do. Do not be reluctant to strike a deal with a colleague on the faculty in a different specialty to exchange items for evaluation.

Obviously, it is also helpful to ask colleagues with the same specialty to read the items. They can validate the content as well as give ideas about what is significant enough to test. Listen to the advice that is given and use it to improve items that need improvement.

Validity of Proficiency Exams

In order to tell whether a proficiency test is doing what it is supposed to do, compare the test performance of people who have not taken the course with the performance of those who have. If the same exam is used in both groups, simply look at the performances of students who enrolled in the course as compared to the performances of the challengers. However, if a different exam is used for the proficiency exam, bias could be introduced that makes the test too hard or too easy compared to what is required of those who enroll.

Student Review of Tests

Students should get feedback on their test grades within a week or so after they take the test. One hotly contested issue about tests is how to give the students feedback about their performance and whether or not to give tests back to students to keep. One reason given for not letting students see their exams is to protect the test-item bank. The other side of this debate is that if the test-item bank is big enough, it does not matter.

If students are able to see their tests without keeping them, schedule a time for students to review the test. Focus on answering questions about rationale, and make the review a learning experience. If the students have complaints, let them put their concerns in writing.

Student feedback can also be provided by having a copy of the exam with the correct answers marked available for them to view at designated times and for a limited time period after the exam. If this method of feedback is used, set some ground rules, such as that the merits of the exam or individual items will not be discussed.

In some schools, tests are routinely given back to students to assist them in their own review. Files of old tests may be maintained and are available to students so that all students have equal access to them, not just those with friends in the previous class. As far as this issue is concerned, it is important to weigh the costs and the benefits of whatever decision you make.

Student Reactions

Feelings always run high about tests. Whenever someone is in a student role, it is tough to be subjected over and over to tests. Because tests frequently constitute a major portion of a course grade, students are concerned about the impact of each test and of each item on their final grades. They can and will argue long and hard for one or two more points. Many teachers are surprised and perplexed about the behavior of students in response to tests.

FINAL WORDS

Testing helps to assess student learning as well as to evaluate teacher success. The procedures in developing items, assembling exams, and analyzing results are complex, but logical. Producing fair tests is a fundamental skill for nursing faculty, but developing that skill takes time and effort.

OTHER RESOURCES YOU WOULD BE WISE TO CONSIDER

Test Construction Workshops

Everyone who writes tests ought to go to a test-construction workshop. These workshops provide a good foundation for constructing tests.

Teaching Centers/Test Review Committee

Many educational institutions have teaching centers, and one of the services provided is assistance in test construction. A staff member can provide a workshop on test construction and evaluation for faculty groups.

Some schools have a test review committee. This committee works with new faculty to enhance their test-construction skills. Also it provides guidance and support to all faculty for test construction issues.

Colleagues

Working with colleagues is an excellent way to improve test-construction skills. Look at colleagues' tests and ask about their judgments. Ask them to evaluate your items.

Course Work

A formal college course may help faculty to write better tests and understand more about the statistics involved. If planning to enroll in such a course, make sure that the content will address your needs. Sometimes courses called "Tests and Measurements" are described in the college catalog as dealing with test construction, but the bulk of the course focuses on statistics.

Educational Testing Service

The Educational Testing Service (ETS) is the leading authority in test development. Many standardized tests used in every level of education and in many professions are developed, printed, or graded by ETS. The service provides consultation to groups who are developing major examinations, such as the American Nurses Association Certification Program. They publish many useful monographs about test construction.

FURTHER READING

McDonald, M. (2002). *Systematic assessment of learning outcomes: Developing multiple choice exams.* Sudbury: Jones & Bartlett.
McKeachie, W. J. (2002). *Teaching tips: Strategies, research, and theory for college university teachers.* (11th ed.). Boston: Houghton Mifflin.

12

Using Technology to Facilitate Learning

Technology encompasses all educational activities that require and involve the use of the computer. The computer is an essential tool for the present-day student. Computers are invaluable for writing papers, collecting and storing class notes, and preparing projects and presentations and for communication with classmates, faculty, and the world. Sometimes the computer may even be the primary source for access to course materials and instruction. Computerized patient-information systems may also be encountered in hospitals, clinics, and other community institutions used for student clinical experience.

GOALS

The principal use of the computer is as a tool to assist students to access, organize, store, retrieve, and communicate information. It may also free faculty from repetitious aspects of teaching and enable a faculty member to become more of a facilitator of learning and communication.

TOOLS

Hardware

Computer

The type of computer is not as important as access to one. Schools often have computer labs or media centers that are available for student use. Because many students may be using the labs, finding a free machine to use may be a problem. A learning resource center is ideal for facilitating faculty and student use of computers. School-wide communication such as conferencing and e-mail is often handled by the use of a local area network (LAN). Students may wish to purchase their own computer to use at home or as a portable on which to take class notes. It is important to inform incoming students of the type of and minimum computer specifications needed for participating in course and school activities. This is essential for students who are planning to participate in distance-learning programs.

Accessories

Media centers and computer or learning labs may be available to provide faculty and students with access to additional hardware accessories, such as videodisk players, slide and presentation projectors, video cameras and monitors, printers, and copy machines. Information regarding hours of operation and the rules and regulations for use of this equipment should be shared with students during orientation. If use of the lab is a requirement for course activities, instructions should be included in the course syllabus.

Software and Applications

Computer programs are available for a wide variety of uses including word processing, database collection, spreadsheets, graphic presentations, and content delivery. Software also comes in different formats including floppy disks, CD-ROMs, videodisks, and licensed networked programs.

Software programs can be used either for class and course-work presentations or for student self-study. Computer-assisted instruction (CAI) programs such as case presentations, simulations, tutorials, and drills may be available in the media center for student self-study. This type of software helps students with specific skills, such as critical thinking, physical assessment, or preparation for NCLEX-RN. Computer-based applications support the needs of students by allowing them to work at their own time and pace and provides for immediate feedback of their progress. Computer programs in the form of floppy disks or CD-ROMs are frequently included with the purchase of required course textbooks. Additional computer program software is available for individual purchase at school or local bookstores. The school may purchase licenses for computer software programs, which are then available for use by both students and faculty on the school's computer local area network (LAN). In this way, these programs can also be accessed from distant sites over modems or dial-in networks. Distance-learning programs use the Internet and World Wide Web for course work and course conferencing. Students and faculty need to become comfortable with the use of basic computer software programs such as word processing as well as database and spreadsheet programs and should have the ability to access the Internet.

NUTS AND BOLTS

Selecting Computer Applications

Process

Using the computer is one method for delivery of course content and evaluation of students' learning. Planning is essential for successful implementation of computer use in the learning process. As with reviewing texts, start by setting the criteria to evaluate options. The methodology and material should be presented in harmony with the rest of the curriculum. Review the program and course objectives to see if there is a good fit. Include the computer-based activities in the course objectives. Try out one new computer methodology per class or course and ask for students' feedback and evaluation. Computer use requires a significant amount of time expenditure and should relate to the course credit. It also should be calculated into both student and faculty workload.

Software Content Evaluation

When assessing software for student self-study, prepare a list of content topics in the course. Be sure the content is covered with emphasis on the aspects considered most important. Also, make sure the software used in the course or for self-study is appropriate for the students. The method and content should be aimed at the level of the student in the class.

Evaluation of computer programs or software for personal use or for purchase by the school computer or media center should occur.

Table 12.1 includes a form that could be used to evaluate CAI software. This form is based on the form used earlier for evaluating a potential textbook (Tables 8.1 and 8.2).

TABLE 12.1 Software Evaluation Form

Name of software_____

Publisher_____

Cost_____

Author_____

Publication date_____

Projected use_____

General:

____ Conceptual framework harmonious with ours

____ Comprehensive coverage of content

____ Emphasis on nursing models

____ Approach to nursing process consistent with ours

____ Definitions consistent with our terminology

____ Builds on prerequisite content

____ Aimed at students in upper division

____ Nonsexist and nonstereotyped language

Usability:

____ User-friendly

____ Clear instructions for getting started and working through the CAI

____ Student can progress at own pace and skip sections if desired

____ Immediate feedback to student

____ Clear instructions for exiting program and student may exit whenever desired

____ Built-in self-assessments or quizzes for students

Support materials:

____ Instructors' manuals available

____ Student manual available

____ Instructions only, not for purchase

____ For individual purchase

    *Cost*____

____ Program-driven media

____ Slides

____ Videodisk

____ Test-item bank available

____ Book form

____ Computer software

Comments:

As with the textbook evaluation, rate the elements with a Likert scale from 0 for "Unsatisfactory" to 5 for "Excellent." Other items may be evaluated simply on the basis of "Yes" or "No."

Costs

The use of technology in instruction requires a significant investment on the part of both the institution and the faculty. Adequate resources must be available to successfully use technology in course presentations. The cost will involve the need for technology support personnel, software, and hardware resources. Investments in resources must be made on an ongoing basis in order for the program to remain technologically current.

Designing Presentations

Numerous programs are available for creating instructional programs and evaluation tools for use with students. One of the most widely used programs for developing classroom presentations is Microsoft PowerPoint. This program can be easily learned and adapted for use in various teaching situations such as classroom and Web-based presentations. More complex computer software authoring systems are also available but require more computer knowledge and expertise.

FINAL WORDS

In this information age it is important to explore the institutional resources that are available to you and to use them to enhance education. In order to help students to be current and competitive as professionals, provide them opportunities to work with computers and show them how to incorporate the use of computers into their professional lives.

FURTHER READING

Adams, A. M. (2004). Pedagogical underpinnings of computer-based learning. *Journal of Advanced Nursing, 46*(1), 5–12.

McConnell, E. A. (2000). High-tech learning means more access, more participation—and more nurses. *Nursing Management, 11,* 49.

13

Guiding Independent Study

Undergraduates in their junior or senior years and graduate students are often ready to study a topic that is not part of the regular curriculum. The names given to these activities vary from one university or college to another and often are called directed readings, special studies, or special topics. Regardless of what they are called, the two basic types of independent study are directed readings and a special activity of some sort, and these are the two types of independent study discussed in this chapter. It is beyond the scope of this book to deal with a major independent study such as a thesis.

Just how independent is independent study? Both the student and faculty member have responsibilities when engaged in independent study. The student is responsible for determining the topic to be addressed and objectives to be accomplished. The faculty member is responsible for helping to provide structure and guidance as well as a format in which the student will receive credit.

GOALS

The principal goal of independent study is to promote autonomy of the student. Independent study helps to provide unique learning experiences that may not be included in the regular curriculum.

TOOLS

Directed Reading

Directed reading involves a student and a faculty member working out a program of reading. Generally, the student identifies a particular area of

TABLE 13.1   A Plan for Directed Reading

Objective: To identify the nursing implications of the use of lithium

Outcomes:

1. Identify side effects and toxic effects of the drug that have implications for nursing supervision of patients.

2. Identify appropriate nursing interventions to be implemented in response to side effects and toxic effects.

3. Make a guide incorporating effects and related interventions.

Activities:

1. Read two to three articles per week.

2. Summarize each article.

3. Meet with faculty member for 2 hours every other week.

Evaluation:

Two hours of credit will be awarded for successfully achieving the outcomes listed above.

Agreed to by:

Student signature_____   Faculty signature_____

---

interest that usually relates to the faculty member's field of expertise. The faculty member guides the student in where to look for appropriate readings in order to meet the student's objectives. (See Table 13.1.)

Special Study

Special studies include all those activities outside of directed reading. This would include observational experiences, clinical practice, and small research studies, among other activities. These activities require faculty to explore unique learning experiences with the student that encourage reflection and analysis of the planned experience. (See Table 13.2.)

NUTS AND BOLTS

Getting Started

Meet with the student to discuss what the student wishes to accomplish. Some students come with very specific ideas about what they want to

TABLE 13.2   A Plan for Special Study

Objectives:

1. To practice facilitating a small group of students learning about group-process concepts
2. To give feedback to promote learning in a small-group experience
3. To modify a structured group experience to meet the needs of the group

Outcomes:

1. Student will be able to describe general principles of promoting healthy group functioning.
2. Student will be able to give constructive feedback to group members.
3. Student will be able to modify group exercises in a way that retains the purpose of the exercises and individualizes the approach to meeting the group's needs.

Activities:

1. Observe a faculty member conducting at least two exercises with a group of junior students.
2. Meet with the faculty member to discuss the process of the group.
3. Conduct four exercises with the group of junior students.
4. Meet with the faculty member prior to each exercise to discuss correct use.
5. Meet with the faculty member after each exercise to discuss group process and progress in meeting outcomes.
6. Read five assignments given by the faculty member.

Evaluation:

Student will meet the outcomes and describe orally to the faculty member how each has been accomplished.

Two hours of credit will be awarded for successfully achieving the outcomes listed previously.

accomplish, whereas others have only a vague notion of what they want. Although you may expect the better students to come with more specific ideas, this is not always the case.

The Student With Specific Ideas

As students progress through their program of study, they may develop a specific interest in a topic, procedure, or drug. When students begin to look into their topics of interest, they may discover there is not much information available in their immediate resources and may become interested in seeking more information. Formation of specific goals and objectives with assistance from faculty will focus this type of inquiry. Activities the student might consider are papers, presentations, facilitation of groups, or clinical preceptorships. After clear goals and objectives are negotiated, a contract between the student and faculty is established. Table 13.1 demonstrates a student–faculty contract for this type of activity.

The Student Without Specific Ideas

Students have many different reasons for choosing independent study. Some may simply need additional credits for graduation or need to be a full-time student. Often they may have only a vague idea at the first meeting of what they need to accomplish. Discussing areas of interest and future plans can help students focus and aid in the decision of whether directed reading or an alternative will best meet their needs.

It is important to spend time with the student narrowing the area for independent study. The activity planned should be structured so that learning is accomplished. Once a plan is made, a formal written contract between the student and faculty will provide a structure for the student. The contract clarifies the ultimate purpose of the activity and the requirements for completion of the independent study. See Table 13.2 for an example of this type of faculty–student contract.

Determination of Credit

In most settings, there is a range of possible credit that may be offered for the categories of independent study. That range usually is one to four credits. Some students request a certain amount of credit, and that should be considered when formulating the plan. Other students do not have a particular amount of credit in mind. During negotiations about the assignment, the student determines the amount of work he or she is willing to put forward, and that will determine the amount of credit.

The school or university may have some stipulations about the amount of time that the student and the faculty member must put into independent study. Check for policies concerning that issue. Such policies should be kept in mind when calculating the amount of work involved in other determinations for credit. It is typical that lecture credit is on the basis of

1 hour of lecture per week for each credit (in a semester system). Clinical and laboratory experiences are usually 3 hours a week for each credit. In addition, there are 2 to 3 hours of preparation or writing outside of class for each credit per week.

Using this information, it would be appropriate to expect the student to devote at least 3 hours a week per credit to the independent study. Part of the initial planning with the student should include making this point so that the student has an adequate idea of the commitment expected. In the case of a directed reading, a consideration when assigning the number of credits may be how long it will take to research the topic adequately. If the student has a certain number of credit hours to fulfill, then the amount of work to achieve that goal should be determined and made clear to the student.

Setting Objectives

The next step is for both student and faculty member to set objectives. Some situations may call for several objectives whereas others may be met with only one or a few objectives.

Approach

After setting objectives, the student and faculty member decide how the student can best achieve his or her learning objectives. In the case of directed reading, in addition to the discussion of evaluation of the objectives, a plan could be made to research and extrapolate the necessary information. In the case of an activity, an agency, case manager, or another faculty member may participate in the student's planned activity.

If a student wants an observational or clinical experience, it may take more time to identify where the student can undertake these experiences. Negotiations with individuals or agencies to permit the student to observe certain activities will be necessary. A careful description of the student's role in the situation must be written; that is, it must be noted that the student is simply to observe and not give patient care.

If a student wants a special clinical experience, work out an appropriate setting for this to take place and provide or arrange for adequate supervision. Providing this sort of independent study is complicated, and the time involved may be too prohibitive to make it possible. An example of this situation would be a student interested in the emergency room. The student could work with a charge nurse or staff nurse who agrees to act as a preceptor. The student would provide care to patients under the supervision of the nurse with the agency's approval. The student could keep a journal, reflecting on the experiences during clinical time, and discuss those experiences with the preceptor. At the end of the student's experience, he or she would submit a final paper or presentation detailing the experience to faculty.

Supervision

The amount of supervision required is determined by the nature of the independent study. Directed reading requires no direct supervision, but it is typical to meet with the student on a regular basis to discuss the readings. With an undergraduate, there is an expectation that summaries of the articles with some higher-level processes will be prepared, such as synthesis or evaluation of the articles. With graduate students, the use of high-level processes should be expected in ways more substantial than simply presenting summaries.

Supervising a special study is more complex and requires more faculty time than supervising directed reading. If the experience is observational, meet regularly with the student to discuss his or her observations and to relate them to the objectives for the experience. With a clinical experience, a faculty member may be directly supervising the student. If the student is assigned to be with a preceptor, meet regularly with the student and plan periodic contacts with the preceptor.

Evaluation

As with all learning experiences, the evaluation is based on the student's ability to meet the objectives that were set. Usually, independent study credit is on a pass-or-fail basis. Even so, the faculty member and the student need to agree on the work that must be completed in order for the student to receive credit. Lack of performance in independent study should be handled as if it were a traditional course. If the student is not doing the work early in the semester, advise the student to drop the course. If the work is not sufficient enough at midterm to indicate to you that the student will be able to complete the work required, give the student a deficiency notice.

In evaluating the actual performance by the student, use the criteria for similar work in other courses. For example, if the student is writing a paper, apply the criteria used in other courses the student may take at the same point in the curriculum. If the student is performing in a clinical setting, expect the same level of performance as in clinical courses at the student's level.

Evaluating students who have participated in predominately observational experiences will depend on the level of objectives that were set. For example, if the student was observing in order to synthesize information, the student would need to demonstrate orally or in writing that this has occurred.

WORDS TO THE WISE

In some academic settings, part of the determination of workload may include credit for the time spent in independent study. Be sure to negotiate for the hours involved when your contract is considered. If you are expected to supervise students in independent study without this being figured into your contracted number of hours, negotiate with your dean or director for release time from other responsibilities such as committee work or some teaching responsibilities. Supervising independent study is not as demanding as some aspects of teaching, but if done right, it takes a lot of time. Be sure to take care of yourself and get credit for it in some way, either in money or in time. The rewards for such an undertaking may be the privilege of observing a student discovering a different career path as a result of the independent study.

FINAL WORDS

Independent study gives students a chance to design learning experiences for themselves. Supervising students in directed readings or other special studies gives faculty a change of pace.

FURTHER READING

Jerlock, M., Falk, K., & Severinsson, E. (2003). Academic nursing education guidelines: Tools for bridging the gap between theory, research and practice. *Nursing and Health Sciences, 5,* 219–228.

Myrick, F., & Yonge, O. (2004). Enhancing critical thinking in the preceptorship experience in nursing education. *Journal of Advanced Nursing, 45*(4), 371–380.

Profetto-McGrath, J. (2003). The relationship of critical thinking skills and critical thinking dispositions of baccalaureate nursing students. *Journal of Advanced Nursing, 43*(6), 569–577.

14

Helping Students Improve Their Writing Skills

Although it is common for nursing instructors to assign papers to meet course requirements, students often are unable to meet the expectations of such assignments. The details about how to design the requirements for a paper as a major assignment are in chapter 9. This chapter deals with how to help students develop writing skills.

College students are generally expected to take one or two courses in English composition. Although these are the courses in which they should learn the basic skills related to grammar and composition, students need continued practice to develop the ability to write effectively. The ideal way to carry this through the nursing major is for the faculty to agree on what kinds of writing their graduates should be able to do and where they need to learn to write what they need to write.

GOALS

The principal goal for helping students to become better writers is to improve their ability to communicate the knowledge they will acquire.

TOOLS

Clear Assignment

To write well, students need to understand what the assignment is. Establish what objectives the students are supposed to meet by the writing assignment. Make clear the important points that the students should address.

Guidelines to Give the Student

Help students improve their writing by giving them some guidance and support in mastering the process of putting ideas on paper. Present these ideas in class or offer an extracurricular time to cover these points.

Preparing to Write

Tell the students to start by outlining the content to be covered. The main topics in the outline will suggest subheadings for the paper. Leave room in the outline to insert additional content as needed. Show them a sample outline. Table 14.1 provides an example of an outline on a specific topic.

Help the students decide how to spend their preparation time in terms of how the assignment will be evaluated. In some assignments, the emphasis is on the content produced. For example, the paper may be a review of the literature on a certain topic.

Other assignments focus on describing a process, such as a nursing-care study. More care may be taken in presenting the content-oriented paper in scholarly tones. On the other hand, a process-oriented paper can be written in the first person.

Practicing Writing

The only way to learn to write is like everything else one learns—practice. Encourage students to start by writing whatever they can think of that fits the writing assignment. Initially, they should not worry about where to start or how the material is organized. As they have ideas for a section, they should start a new page and write what they are thinking. After they have written for a while, they should leave their written work alone for a few days. When they read it again, they may see grammatical errors or problems in composition they overlooked when it was fresh. Then they should rewrite the paper cleaning up the errors, with more attention to grammar and organization. As they read more about the topic, they will have more ideas for what they are writing. They should set it aside again for a few days.

Although what they have written may still seem rough, they are ready to ask someone else to read it. Reading drafts of the students' papers is time-consuming, but it may be possible to allocate time to read at least a page or two of each one. Reading the drafts gives faculty indications

TABLE 14.1 Outline for Writing a Paper

Clients Who Split: Borderline Personality Disorder

1. Introduction

   a. Childhood disruptions

      Inconsistent parenting

      Promotion of negative self-concept

   b. Characteristics

      Impulsive

      Manipulative

   c. Internal conflicts

      Clinging/distancing

      Dependence/independence

2. Problems for nursing intervention

   a. Acting-out behavior: sexual promiscuity, substance abuse, temper tantrums, suicidal threats and gestures

   b. Manipulative behavior: splitting, blaming, helplessness

   c. Relationship behavior: "yo-yoing," clinging, distancing

   d. Impulsive behavior: running away

3. Nursing interventions

   a. Firm, consistent, positive attitude

   b. Expect appropriate behavior

   c. Foster development of trust

   d. Constructive confrontation

   e. Encourage verbalization of feelings

   f. Reinforce efforts at individuation

   g. Set firm limits on manipulation

   h. Teach coping with reality problems

   i. Maintain frequent, open communication among staff to provide consistent approach

4. Description of client with examples

5. Summary

about the students' progress and provides the opportunity to give students some constructive suggestions for improving their papers before they get to the last draft.

They may also ask other people to read and critique what they wrote. They should explain why they are practicing and provide the ground rules for how much feedback they really want. However, to gain as much as they can from the experience, they should give their readers as much latitude as possible to critique the work. They should ask their readers not only to say what they do not like but also to provide some suggestions.

Coping with Negative Experiences

With a lot of difficult experiences, students become discouraged because they are not totally successful the first time they try. Some of this is a legacy of "learning experiences" they had in the past when faculty members criticized them for not doing better when they tried a new skill for the first time—or at least it felt like criticism.

After freshman English courses, nursing students usually have no courses requiring formal writing. Then, suddenly, they are in one of their major courses, and they not only have to convey information about what they did for a patient, but have to convey it skillfully as well. Because they have not been practicing this skill, they may have forgotten a lot of what they learned.

NUTS AND BOLTS

Guidelines for Writing Well

Use these suggestions to assist students with improving their writing skills.

Guidelines for better writing:

1. Make and follow an outline.
2. Use simple declarative sentences.
3. When in doubt about how something sounds, throw it out.
4. Avoid pretentious touches such as literary quotations that do not advance the reader's understanding of your subject.
5. Avoid slang and other colloquialisms.
6. Stop once the point is made.

7. Usually a cumbersome, ambiguous, or confusing sentence can be improved by one of the following methods: (a) break it up into more than one sentence, (b) shorten it rather than add to it, or (c) drop it altogether.
8. Use the same tense throughout unless there is a particular reason to do otherwise.
9. Make sure the subject and verb of each sentence agree in number.
10. Avoid sexist language.
11. Use the third person in formal papers unless the situation calls for a first-person account.
12. Start writing and putting ideas together without worrying about how it sounds. Polish it later after getting down the gist of the ideas and points.
13. After writing something, leave it alone for a few days. Then reread it and polish it.
14. If you are unsure of the spelling of a word, look it up in the dictionary. Spell-check your finished document if using the computer.
15. The greater the sense of accomplishment upon completing the first draft of a work, the greater the need for revision.
16. If experiencing trouble writing a first sentence, start somewhere else.
17. If experiencing trouble writing a last sentence, you have probably already written it.
18. Write something every day, even if it is not directly related to your major writing project.
19. Do not be afraid to let someone read and edit the paper. Make sure the person has the expertise to critique the content and style.
20. Get one or two handbooks on English (not texts) to help answer questions about syntax, grammar, and usage.
21. Use the computer. It makes the process much easier for most people.
22. Break up your piece with headings, subheadings, and so on. Use underlining and italics for emphasis.
23. If using references, make bibliography cards on all articles, books, and personal interactions as soon as you get them, even if you may not use them. Write your citation of the source in the same style you intend to use for the finished product. Use of a computer program to manage the references is highly recommended. This makes management of the literature and citation of references along with the reference page of the paper much easier and more manageable.

Critiquing Writing

When evaluating your students' written work, be as constructive as possible. Sensitivity to students' vulnerability as feedback is provided is crucial. Advise them that developing this important skill is vital for their future in nursing while reassuring them that mastery of this skill is attainable through practice.

FINAL WORDS

Writing effectively is a useful skill for nurses. Because nursing education occurs within institutions of higher learning, part of the major is becoming a well-rounded person as well as a skillful nurse. Nursing faculty members can offer a lot to students by helping them to overcome some of their negative attitudes about expressing themselves in writing.

FURTHER READING

American Psychological Association. (2001). *Publication manual of the American Psychological Association* (5th ed.). Washington, DC: Author.
Strunk, W. (2000). *The elements of style* (4th ed.). Longman: New York.

Index

Page numbers in italic indicate tables.